VIRTUAL
MEDICINE

These new concepts of life and energy bring back a medicine
of humility before the miracle we call life. The art of medicine becomes a practice composed of the life energies of the
physician, the patient and the Earth.

Dr Robert O. Becker, *Cross Currents: The Perils of
Electropollution, The Promise of Electromedicine*

By the same author:

The Complete Guide to Food Allergy and Environmental Illness

Food Allergy Plan

The Allergy Handbook

Allergies: What Everyone Should Know

Diet Wise: Let Your Body Choose The Food That's Right For You

VIRTUAL MEDICINE

A new dimension in energy healing

Dr. Keith Scott-Mumby

MB ChB, MD, PhD, FCRP *(Medicina Alternativa)*

Polimedia Communications Publishers

To Telly, who saw the dark hour when it was conceived,
and was there in the happy hour it was born.

Publishers:
Polimedia Communications
78-015 Main Street, Suite 204
La Quinta, CA 92253
USA

10 9 8 7 6 5 4 3 2 1

A catalogue record for this book is available from the British Library
and from the Library of Congress, Washington

ISBN 978-0-9768617-2-0

Printed in USA by
Bang Printing, 3323 Oak Street, Brainerd, MN 56401

Contents

	Foreword – Preface	*vi*
1	Join the Party, Doc	1
2	The History of Energy Medicine	17
3	Biology Beyond the Skin	33
4	The Birth of Electro-Acupuncture	53
5	The Vegatest	73
6	Bioresonance Therapy	91
7	Basic Treatment Modalities	107
8	Electro-Dermal Computer Screening	133
9	Light as Therapy	153
10	Gaia	171
11	Star Trek Medicine is Here... Now!	187
12	Weird or What?	201
13	The Non-Material Nature of Substances	217
14	Biology Beyond Death	237
15	Electronic Kundalini	251
	Resources	267
	Index	275

FOREWORD

There are books which are ahead of their time and books which do not break new ground in terms of recent intellectual developments. But, once in a while, a book like *Virtual Medicine* comes along which is truly pivotal.

Keith Scott-Mumby has managed to tread a careful path through the domain of esoteric, metaphysical matters, throwing light on the case and yet not being bogged down by the associated mystical rhetoric. His story reads like an 'adventure' into knowledge and is underpinned with frequent sound scientific references. In this way, Keith has pushed the cause of holism and integrated medicine considerably beyond its previous perameters.

Werner Heisenberg, one of the founders of modern quantum physics, said: *the most fruitful developments in human history have come when two different lines of thought have met*. Such 'lines' may have their roots in quite different parts of human culture, in different times, different intellectual environments and alien religions but they may nevertheless interact and produce new and exciting developments.

This seems to be the case with the Virtual Medicine paradigm. It is the meeting of Eastern philosophical healing systems and Western technological science which has led to a most fruitful advance. Chinese and Ayurvedic models are based on the wisdom that the body possesses a natural ability to resist disease and heal itself, when correctly stimulated; only now are we able to work scientifically with these esoteric disciplines using new technology.

Virtual Medicine both looks back over the ground we have conquered and forward with clarity and discernment into the future and where we are going. It is stimulating to the mind and intellect, well researched and written in accord with established medical parameters. I would wish to see it widely read, especially by our more conventional colleagues, and furthermore see this journey from metaphysics and philosophy to quantum physics and scientific realism adopted as tomorrows mainstream medical thinking and practise.

Professor (Dr.med) Michael F. Kirkman

PREFACE

I hope the revelations in Virtual Medicine will fascinate and delight the reader with new insights into age-old questions of disease, vitality and even death. It would fail if it did not at least shock some. You will see, in the chapters to come, that certain practitioners are able to detect life events beyond the confines of the body. That is to say that real-time phenomena, which once would of appeared magical, occult or 'etheric', can be identified using ordinary scientific equipment tuned to do so, devices which I have labelled as belonging to the domain of Virtual Medicine (or cyber-healing). If nothing else, this shows us that life is not merely a property of physical matter.

You will also learn that disease as we now know it is nothing more than the final result of events which have been going on in and around the body for a long period before anything is noticeably wrong. Once again, we can now witness these danger events in real-time, using advanced equipment to visualize them, and this opens up the possibility of successful 'treatment' before ever the disease manifest. Here is another reason for using the term Virtual Medicine. It is healing at a higher and more intelligent dimension.

There is some discussion about what was called, earlier this century, the new physics - meaning the startling revelations of quantum mechanics and Einstein's mind-bending principles of Relativity. Add to that the powerful assertion of chaos as a governing principle of the dynamics we actually experience. Gradually science has had to adopt a new view of reality that was not much to its liking.

Einstein's famous equation, $e = mc2$, has caused us to modify our view of particles and matter in a essential way. We had to start thinking of matter or 'stuff' as a property of energy. This means that matter can no longer be viewed as something static or permanent. It is equivalent to a certain amount of energy or process, which expresses itself in the form of something apparently tangible.

Then in almost contemporaneous development quantum mechanics came along, with its strange sub-atomic world of probability and 'virtual particles' from the great quantum field. Particles just leapt into existence in this void and vanished again just as adroitly. Physics was beginning to sound more like witchcraft than science.

Then suddenly in the last quarter-century of this millennium we have discovered that our 'advanced physics' is beginning to meet ancient systems of the mind, such as Tao and the Vedas. That is to say, science is catching up with older wisdom, not the other way round. There is a remarkable and quite stirring concordance between texts written thousands of years ago and what scientists working at the leading edge of knowledge are discovering about today's reality.Despite this swing of emphasis and broadening of philosophy in the leading natural science of physics, medicine has consistently refused to tune in to the important new issues. If only doctors knew more physics they probably would not rant and rail against healing alternative disciplines quite as much as they do like to. Chemistry, biology and other disciplines all necessarily take their cues from physics, but not medicine, seemingly. Instead those doctors who wished to establish better healing values in this new domain were attacked, quite savagely at times, and denounced vituperatively as charlatans and snake-oil peddlers.

Well I'm pleased to say that things have begun to change. We are seeing a rebirth of the philosophy of Vitalism, the understanding that the world we experience is structured and takes its cues from life itself. Not from some meaningless clockwork motor which God or somebody installed 'at the beginning' and has run ever since. Life is no longer some menace that got into the perfect machine but is the creator of all. It is a living and conscious universe where energy and dynamic process are the basis of reality.

We now have a better and more functional model of health and disease. The age of energy medicine is here.

Dr Keith Scott-Mumby

Marbella 1999

www.alternative-doctor.com

www.dietwisebook.com

www.askdoctorkeith.com

CHAPTER 1

JOIN THE PARTY, DOC

Our view of the world is changing fast. A quarter of a century ago there were things that scientists were absolutely *certain* were true which, today, we are absolutely certain are *not true*. Nowhere is this more evident than in the physics of organisms. In just a few decades we have moved from the position where the human energetic aura was deemed not to exist, to the point where there is ample scientific proof of its existence and several good theories as to its nature and function. Studies have been carried out in many major universities of the world which, although they are largely ignored by those who have some other 'truth' to peddle, have nevertheless done a great deal to unite realms that were once held to be only metaphysical (hence the name) with the accepted tenets of everyday science. We now have instruments which can measure effects on this order of reality; what is emerging is that the truth has indeed been out there a *long* time.

Nobody was really paying attention.

Until this recent era of enquiry into biological energy, any belief in the aura or psychokinetic effects was considered to be a childish construct of less scientific (and therefore mistaken) peoples; the typical view of our Western boffins was that what these peoples lacked in sophisticated understanding of reality they made up for in myths and 'mumbo-jumbo'. Shamans were just witch-doctors, and hands-on healing was a fraud that relied on self-delusion by gullible souls.

The mere fact that some of these supposedly naïve beliefs have been around for thousands of years, compared to a few centuries of our science, does not seem to carry any weight with those guilty of this hubris. Yet the reality is that science, as its own proponents define it, is a shifting quicksand of fashions and opinions, which regularly contradicts itself – often embarrassingly so.

Two of the grandest and most revolutionary theories of the last century, Einstein's Relativity and Planck's quantum mechanics, are in such disharmony that they appear mutually exclusive. The Big Bang hypothesis of cosmology has all but collapsed due to inconsistencies, according to Professor Andrei Linde at California's Stanford University, though those who make their living writing about it refuse to admit there are major discrepancies, and march on blindly as if nothing were wrong.[1] It is a disconcerting fact that electricity and magnetism, two of the absolutely fundamental building blocks of the universe, are so little understood that, at the deepest level, science cannot explain the nature of these energetic phenomena or how they exert their effect. We recognize the electron as a basic building block, which has properties, such as mass and charge, but a deeper explanation of how these properties arise is lacking.

I make this point in case the reader is under the illusion that science, in any meaningful sense, understands our world. It doesn't.

My greatest complaint with so-called science is not that it is sometimes wrong but that it fails to acknowledge that whenever something cannot be shown to exist using the standard narrow approach, it is labelled 'unscientific' and therefore a fake or delusion. There is never any suggestion that the problem may be the fault of science or its inadequate methodology. Yet 120 years ago there was no way to detect radio waves. Did that mean they were an 'unscientific' belief, if anyone had come up with the idea ahead of its time? Even more importantly, could it be said that because the science of the day failed to detect such a phenomenon *that therefore radio waves did not exist?*

THE REBIRTH OF VITALISM

Philosophers speak of an epistemology of 'naïve realism'; it means thinking that all you see is all there is. Very naïve.

Yet modern mechanistic science is stuck in this frame of mind. It is predicated wholly on the belief that there is nothing more to our experience of Being than a heap of matter which (supposedly) came into existence ready-formed in some giant flash at the start of time. The irony of this is that Isaac Newton, who fathered this view of the world, was himself deeply embroiled in the occult, magic, alchemy and other mystical matters which today's scientist effects to despise and ridicule. Of course it is Newton's followers who have gone over the edge into the legitimacy of this so-called 'clockwork' universe. The dismay of his biographers in trying to reconcile the man as they wanted to see him and the truth of his past led to the virtual suppression of most of his writings – 'The obvious production of a fool and a knave,' as one of his biographers described this secret material.[2]

In the 20th century we have been forced to look again at the mechanistic universe and, finally, brave new writers like Rupert Sheldrake are coming out with a refreshing paradigm, which is that life and the conscious process make matter, and not the other way round.[3] The model of the world in which the energies of life are pre-eminent and drive creation is called *Vitalism*.

One of the greatest proponents of this philosophy was Henri Bergson (1859–1941), who received the Nobel Prize for literature in 1927 and became a member of l'Académie Française (1941). He is author of *Matter and Memory* (1896) and *Creative Evolution* (1907). Sir John C. Eccles, (1903–1997) the distinguished Australian neurophysiologist and 1963 Nobel laureate, expounds his version of Vitalism in *Evolution of the Brain: Creation of the Self*.[4] Vitalism is the traditional view of the world, eclipsed briefly for a few centuries under the weight of scientific excesses, but now forcing itself upon us as the only truth which can explain what we see – no fudging.

Of course it would be wrong to try and remove the word 'science' from the dictionary of common-sense. But science needs rehabilitating from the pompous and pedantic position it has taken and made into what it should be: the discipline of knowledge and learning *all the truth*. In the fullest sense, science, philosophy and religion come together. There can be no science that violates the precepts of sacredness and Being, attempting to dismiss life as some weird accident in the chemical machine.

INFORMATION FIELDS

The newest concept in biology is the *information field*. Information fields create reality; they put it there and hold it together the way it should be. Have you ever wondered why a teacup is a teacup? Why don't the atoms at the edge go wandering off and become, say, a spoon? The answer is an information field. When you drink a cup of tea you do so from something which, in material terms, is 99.999999 per cent not there (please don't count the decimal places, there are dozens I didn't bother to type). Only the field is real. Matter, as quantum physics teaches us, is a mere illusion. It comes out of this 'void' or vacuum, whenever we interact with it. Like the cavalry troops in the old B movies, it shows up just when it's needed!

It follows that a cancer, a parasite or a virus are also just information fields. Everything in our life and being is energy and information. We come from fields in the egg; we go back to a field as a corpse. Indeed, there is the likelihood that we survive death at least as some kind of field.

Biological information fields are unbelievably vast in the amount of data which they contain —- many orders of magnitude greater than the combined total molecular complexity of our physical substances. In other words, there is no way that the biochemical plasma of our bodies could contain enough information to organize and control a living organism. We need the information field to put us there and hold us in place. Chemicals cannot 'think' and organize other chemicals without some initiating input! This one fact really does put paid once and for all to the idea of biochemically-based life, as espoused by the current drug-based medical culture. We exist as regulated and informed energy.

According to 1984 Nobel Laureate Carlo Rubbia, matter ('stuff') is less than a billionth part of the manifest cosmos. The rest is pure energy phenomena of interaction, information fields and resonance. This is a staggering revelation, from one of science's top minds. A healing discipline which looks only at such a tiny and inconsequential part of the whole is badly skewed, and is bound to get it wrong more often than right. Stuck in the incorrect 'matter' paradigm, ignorant doctors are surely doomed to violate the first precept of Hippocrates' code, which is: 'Do no harm.'

Unfortunately, doctors are decades behind with this and are not even talking about the idea yet. Scientific attitudes here, I am sorry to say, are often no more than an affectation with which the medical establishment tries to brow-beat its (many) opponents, rather than the humble reality of willing seekers of truth. It is a case where, as the founder of humanistic psychology Abram Maslow put it, the pretence of science is being used to avoid the bigger truth.

FIELD DISTURBANCES

Remember that information implies consciousness of a sort. It is inescapable. David Pearson, with his theories of the 'living universe' (conscious matter), has found remarkable success and accord among physics and mathematical colleagues. But once again the doctors were not at the party![5]

It is interesting to note that the word information means to give material form to (from the Latin: *informare*). In other words, information at the quantum field level is actually an active, creative force intimately involved in the form and manifestation of reality. Stated differently, information is a specific way of representing the interaction of consciousness and reality, either as a means of organizing it or decoding it. It is too early to be sure *how* these fields operate and influence things, except to say that quantum probability fields seem the intermediate domain between consciousness and reality made manifest. Even without a full understanding, it is a major paradigm shift to recognize they are there and the critical role they play.

Disease can now be redefined as a disruption, cessation or distortion arising in the information and energy fields. The *best* way to approach disease then, surely, is by correcting these disturbances, which will then eliminate the disharmony and disease process – in other words, bring about healing.

We call this **Energy Medicine** (sometimes vibrational medicine) and it is a theme which is central to the material in this book.

If virtual reality means virtual fields, and virtual matter springs from virtual energy, then it's time we gave up the whole idea of the importance of material substances and started to think differently about our world. As soon as we do so, the world begins to take on a spiritual, almost metaphysical reality, and religious factors enter into the equation. As Dr. Richard Gerber, author of *Vibrational Medicine*, says, 'The unseen connection between the physical body and the subtle forces of spirit holds the key to understanding the inner relationship between matter and energy. When scientists begin to comprehend the true relationship between matter and energy, they will come closer to understanding the relationship between humanity and God.'[6]

Healing, then, becomes a loving matter of bringing to the distressed part or organism some kindly or enfolding energy or resonance which soothes the disharmony and coaxes forth healing, instead of violently suppressing the symptoms, which are only manifestations of the body's 'fight-back' response. This healing method is both more rational and more effective, since manifestly we are going further 'upstream' to treat and cure. In fact if we go far enough towards the source, we inevitably encounter the mystery and might of consciousness itself.

The role of consciousness in health and disease has yet to be grasped by the average physician, but it is impossible to leave it to mystics and theological scholars. The nature of life and Being is the key to the door of healing! I believe consciousness is a kind of creative energy force and that, whether we understand it or not, we need to try and work towards incorporating it in our model of health and disease. Life is an expression of this consciousness, as the shamans have been telling us.

DULL TUMMY, NOT SO DULL RESEARCH

At the start of the 20th century, distinguished American neurologist Albert Abrams observed something remarkable, though for all his life he was totally unable to explain it. The man was no intellectual lightweight and had studied conventional medicine with the best doctors of the time in Europe – Virchow, Wasserman, Helmholz and others – winning top honours and a gold medal from Heidelberg University. You can be sure he knew what he was seeing, even if he couldn't understand it.

Abrams returned to the US and taught pathology at Stanford University's medical school in California. One day, when he was percussing (tapping on) the abdomen of a patient with his fingers, the resonant note went suddenly dull. It coincided with the moment when a nearby x-ray machine was switched on. But what was remarkable was that when Abrams rotated the patient, he found the dull note was only present when the patient was oriented east—west. It was a spectacular example of science from a serendipitous moment, where the prepared mind, in the right place at the right time, observes something which everyone else would surely miss.

Subsequently, during a routine examination of a patient suffering from cancer (of the lip), Abrams noticed the same strange dull percussion note when tapping certain areas of the abdomen. It turned up on other cancer patients and tuberculosis cases, but again only if the body was aligned with feet towards the west. Abrams subsequently found this dullness in healthy cases when they were merely in close proximity to cancer or tuberculosis specimens and, most astonishing of all, in cases where the patient was remote from the pathological disease specimen but connected to it by means of a wire.[7]

Abrams' conclusion, quite logically, was that unknown waves were being emitted by diseased tissue and that these could produce physical alteration within the body. He went on to find that he could pass a metal disc over the patient's body, connected to the wire, and when he came to the site of pathology the note would again go dull. When a sceptical colleague challenged him to find the exact location of a tuberculous infection of the lung, Abrams did so accurately. He was able to repeat this numerous times in different cases and with uncanny accuracy.

Abrams went on to develop an instrument he called the *Reflexophone* as a means of detecting and quantifying the strange radiation. A variable resistance altered the current and the machine emitted a sound which varied in pitch, thus eliminating the need to percuss the abdomen. He spoke in terms of differing 'rates' for each disease process and compiled a disease register: 55 for syphilis, 58 for sarcomatous tissue, and so on. Even when testing blind, he could infallibly detect or 'diagnose' disease tissue, using his device. Even more incredibly, Abrams found that by adding new resistors to the Reflexophone, he could calibrate the device in such a way it would say how far advanced the disease process was!

Finally, as if to annoy his conventional colleagues to the extreme, Abrams announced that he could dispense with the patient's physical presence altogether and use only a spot of the subject's blood, hair or urine for testing. Not only that, but he could obtain his 'electronic reactions' by having a healthy subject point to the part of their own body which was diseased in the patient, while connected to the Reflexophone. It was all too fantastic to believe.

One day, while Abrams was demonstrating to a class the reaction produced by the blood of a malaria patient, he went one stage further. The known treatment of malaria was quinine, an alkaloid from the bark of the Cinchona tree. Abrams put a few grains of quinine sulphate into the test tray, together with the malarial blood and, to everyone's amazement, the dull percussion note vanished. The reaction was cancelled out. Other known antidotes behaved similarly; for example, mercurial salts for syphilis. With the insight of genius, Abrams suggested there were unknown radiations emitted by the quinine molecule which *exactly* cancelled out the emanations from the malaria specimen.

From this he reasoned, logically, that it should be possible to build a machine which could broadcast electrical oscillations at just the right counter-frequency, and thereby alter the characteristics of diseased tissue and effect a cure.

Virtual Medicine was on the way!

In co-operation with Samuel O. Hoffman, a radio research engineer who had distinguished himself in the First World War by devising an early form of radar to detect approaching German zeppelins at a great distance, Abrams came up with his *Oscilloclast*. It did indeed offer some remarkable cures. His ideas began to spread and shake the foundations of the medical establishment. In his prophetic words, 'As physicians we dare not stand aloof from the progress made in physical science and segregate the human entity from other entities of the physical universe.'

However, conventional science was not ready for this new wisdom.

VILIFICATION
Predictably, Abrams was attacked by orthodoxy. When he perhaps unwisely announced in 1922 that he had used his instruments to successfully diagnose a patient over telephone wires, he was quickly denounced as a quack in the *Journal of the American Medical Association*.

When the *British Medical Journal* repeated the scurrilous and defamatory attack, Sir James Barr, past president of the British Medical Association, wrote furiously in defence of Abrams:

'You [BMJ] very seldom quote from the Journal of the American Medical Association and one might have expected that when you did you would have chosen a more serious subject than an ignorant tirade against an eminent medical man, against, in my opinion, the greatest genius in the medical profession.'

Abrams died in 1924. The vituperation continued for some time, including 18 consecutive issues of *Scientific American*. One of the worst insinuations was that Abrams had no scientific motive but was merely trying to make money by gulling an unsuspecting community. In truth, Abrams, son of a rich San Francisco merchant, had inherited a vast fortune and was a millionaire in his own right. He had written to Upton Sinclair, the American writer and journalist, offering to donate his devices and work *unpaid* for any institute which would develop the 'Abrams Box' for the benefit of humanity.

Such is the integrity of medical journalism.

THE EMANOMETER
There is another twist to the enthralling story, in which the truth fared a little better. It is worth telling in brief, since it is important to the credibility of the Virtual Medicine paradigm. In 1922 a British homeopathic physician, Dr. William Boyd, built a modified

version of the Oscilloclast called an Emanometer, and confirmed all Abrams' findings. Boyd was a keen researcher, particularly in the field of electro-physics, and he published extensive scientific physiological and biochemical research. He presented a very detailed paper on the workings of the Emanometer at the International Homeopathic Conference in London in 1927. As well as diagnosing, Boyd used it to test homeopathic remedies and let the instrument choose a suitable similimum (for a full account of homeopathy and Virtual Medicine, see Chapter 7). It was quite successful by all accounts — but it was all so startling that controversy was, of course, inevitable.

Accordingly, in 1924 a committee was set up by the Royal Society of Medicine to investigate Boyd's claims, under the chairmanship of Sir Thomas Horder (later Lord Horder). The results were reported to the Royal Society of Medicine in January 1925. It is little short of astonishing that Horder found the Emanometer and percussion method quite valid; over the space of years I pay respect to his integrity. One would have expected official fudging. The fact is, all the committee members were able to detect the change in percussion note first described by Abrams, and the detector apparatus was considered to offer important new diagnostic possibilities. In a series of 25 trials, Boyd's method was shown to be 100 per cent accurate, identifying chemicals and tissues presented in a manner which was 'indistinguishable by visual or other normal' means.[8]

THE BLACK BOX AND RADIONICS

Unfortunately, the committee made no cogent recommendations for further research, and since neither they nor Boyd had the faintest idea how the equipment might work, the Black Box was subsequently ignored and passed into medical history. It now stands as a watchword for humbug and pseudo-science among the sceptics. However, this story is far from ended, as later chapters on electro-acupuncture and electro-dermal screening with a modern computer will reveal.

Meanwhile, George de la Warr in Britain and Ruth Drown in the US had devised their own versions of Abrams' instrument, and for a time considerable interest began to develop in radiesthesia or radionics, as their new technique became known. However, the enthusiasts were to remain entirely outside the medical profession and detector instruments were soon being sold to all and sundry, most of whom had no legal medical qualifications. Inevitably bizarre, exaggerated or just stupid interpretations were being made which soon brought the whole system into grave disrepute.

The catastrophic and manifestly unjust imprisonment of Ruth Drown for supposed fraud shattered any remaining credibility and heralded the end of any chance for the new medicine to slip into mainstream practice (she had been tricked by use of a spot of chicken blood on which she had passed a 'diagnosis'). Radionics limps on, staunchly defended by a few nobly-indignant devotees but hardly taken seriously, even by most fringe practitioners. It has been unable to shake off the stigma of its shaky beginnings and the criminal indictment of its principal founder.

BIOLOGICAL RESONANCE

The key question here is: 'What scientific effect had Abrams found?' It might be argued that one or two paid practitioners were fraudsters; but members of a UK Government committee were hardly likely all to be stooges. They had seen *something* credible, after all. Can we put a name to it after all this time? I believe the answer is an unqualified 'Yes', and it is not magic moonbeams or alien rays.

Abrams himself discovered a clue. While he was in Naples he watched the famous tenor Enrico Caruso flick a wine glass to produce its note or tone and then, by singing the same note, shatter the glass. We call this phenomenon *resonance*. You can try it for yourself in the bathtub; simply sing or hum a higher and higher note and at some point you will hear a loud booming effect where the loudness of the sound is markedly enhanced. At this exact pitch your voice is resonating with the basic wavelength of the room, according to its size (the smaller the room, the higher the resonance note).

In my view, the so-called Abrams' reflex was a spectacular example of the principle of *cyclotron resonance*, though demonstrated over half a century before this important magnetic phenomenon was recognized and explained. With the discovery of the cyclotron resonance effect, advanced physics is almost ready to shake hands with energy healing and telepathy. It is critical to the understanding of the functioning of most of the remarkable new diagnostic and therapy systems in the chapters which follow.

Nobel Prize double-nominee Robert O. Becker tells us, 'The electromagnetic resonance concept may provide an intriguing link to a number of little understood and disputed phenomena, such as extrasensory perception and the ability of "healers" to diagnose and treat patients. In both these activities, the participants may be unconsciously using an innate biological mechanism similar to that of magnetic-resonance imaging (MRI).'[9]

Everyone today is familiar with MRI, though usually without necessarily comprehending the technicalities involved. In principle it isn't difficult, though of course the reality may be far more involved than we know. A charged particle or chemical 'ion', when in a fixed magnetic field such as the earth's own field, is made to spin; the stronger the magnetic effect, the faster the spin. Each atomic substance has different spin characteristics.

If a second oscillating (ON—OFF) field is applied, at an angle of (exactly) 90 degrees to the original field, then the spin motion is enhanced according to the principle we call resonance; it is the same effect as piano or violin strings beginning to hum in sympathy with musical notes of the right frequency sounded nearby. The particles *gain* energy. If the field is suddenly interrupted, the particles give up this extra energy, which is radiated outwards (Figure 1). An image can be formed by placing the body in a fixed field and then bombarding it with an oscillating field, flowing at right angles. When the oscillating field is ON, the ions pick up energy; when the oscillating field is OFF, the ions re-radiate the energy in a form which can be picked up and displayed on a computer as a three-dimensional image. That's really all there is to MRI.

Cyclotron Resonance

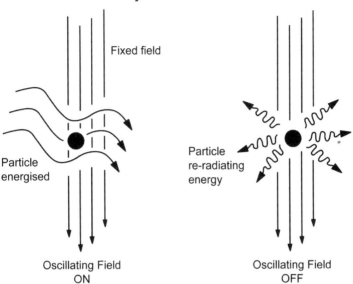

Fixed field

Particle
energised

Particle
re-radiating
energy

Oscillating Field
ON

Oscillating Field
OFF

The enhanced energy effect we call cyclotron resonance. What is important is that the weaker the static field, the smaller the oscillating cross-field needed to create the resonance effect.

To be exact, the non-local effect that would best explain Abrams' findings is nuclear magentic resonance (NMR). Whereas cyclotron resonance is a phenomenon of classical physics, nuclear magentic resonance belongs to the strange world of quantum physics.

RATS ON PARADE

It is impossible to over-estimate the biological importance of this magnetic resonance effect. Living forms exist within the Earth's field, which is very weak. Thus only the slightest disturbance, if at the right frequency and in the critical direction, could have profound effects on important ions such as calcium, sodium and potassium (note how Abrams' reflex *only* operated if the body was oriented feet to the West). It is only a matter of time before scientists begin to wonder if certain diseases are not becoming more common because the typical fields we experience are the ones which interfere with the ordered metabolism of critical ions (the rise in osteoporosis, which depends on functioning levels of calcium ions, is an example I have in mind).

To show how easily this could come about, consider an experiment carried out at the US Naval Research Center, Bethesda, Maryland, and published in the journal *Biomagnetics* in 1986. In this study the effects of cyclotron magnetic resonance on lithium in rat brains was monitored, using a fixed field of 0.2 gauss (low end of the Earth's field strength) and an oscillating field of 60 Hz, which is the frequency of the US domestic mains supply. The reasoning was that if the lithium was truly enhanced by the magnetic resonance effect, then the rats should display more subdued behaviour, since lithium is known as a central nervous system depressant. In fact the rats were exposed to:

- the 60 Hz field alone
- lithium frequency alone
- a combined oscillating and lithium field
- a sham (null) field

Unexposed controls were used, as part of standard scientific protocol.[10]

In due course, it was obvious that the rats exposed to cyclotron resonance were indeed significantly subdued. This result was the equivalent of giving the rats a substantial dose of lithium; in fact they had been given none. The study is important because it shows major biological effects with low-strength fields acting on chemical substances common within the body. It also shows that fields in a typical home are significant biologically. In fact we worry a great deal these days about the particular frequencies between 10 and 100 Hz. These are considered extremely-low-frequency, or ELF, fields. The US military is seeking to develop weapons and population control using this type of radiation. It may be less destructive than nuclear warfare, but such abuse of scientific knowledge is reprehensible and very sinister.

One can only hope that the fools who have sanctionered this idea are not the same people likely to give the order for its use, otherwise God help us all.

RESONANCE IN THE HEALING CONTEXT

You may be sure that the military does not involve itself in phenomena which are illusory (other than the general case of trying to 'win' a war by killing people and destroying material goods). On the contrary, the military is often responsible for important new advances in technology, such as radar, jet engines and space rockets. In time, these new concepts in the physical sciences will filter into the medical model, bypassing the Galenite die-hards, and create what will surely be a major paradigm shift. Hopefully, research will rapidly advance and what many practising therapists from a number of holistic disciplines have known for years will be found to have a credible scientific footing. It is a constant lament of mine that if only doctors knew more advanced physics, they would be less inclined to attack alternative healing.

Experiments using the newest scientific test devices, such as the SQUID magnetometer (see Chapter 2), have shown conclusively that hands-on healers are able to generate a magnetic field around their hands. Couple this fact with the presence of the Earth fixed magentic field and it can be readily seen that the ideal conditions for magnetic resonance are present.

A skilled healer merges his or her whole body field with that of the patient. It is entirely possible, indeed probable, that these healers interact on the resonance principle and create effects which, though we do not understand them properly, begin to fit with known measured reality.

Even 'faith healing' may not be a matter of faith, after all.

ENERGY BEING

We have now reached the stage where we can sensibly postulate life as an energy Being which is manifest in the presence of a body or organism but is definitely *not* confined to the physical structure concerned. This energy presence is a source for wholesome good in the organism but may, due to various reasons yet little understood, become corrupted or disturbed and so give off harmful emanations which act upon the body organism and result in the disease process. The way is open for many legitimate healing techniques which can diagnose using these energy changes, and cause beneficial modifications of the energy forces. I have termed this concept **Virtual Medicine**, since nothing is done in the material domain. Only the results are felt there. Everything takes place in a super-ordinate world of information and energy.

What has stimulated this book is the recognition that the world of high-tech medicine and cutting-edge physics is beginning to drift markedly in the direction of alternative development streams in healing. There is equipment we shall be reviewing which has been around even longer than CAT scanners and MRI, which can tell us a great deal about the health and biological status of a human being. In the chapters to follow we will be looking at systems which can:

- 'listen' for the transmission of pathogens from the tissues
- detect old and unresolved diseases which can affect our present health
- tell electronically whether disease is psychosomatic
- sense the development of cancer as an energy field *years* before it actually becomes manifest as a disease entity.

We are entering a totally new world-view where electronics, quantum physics and the computer meet age-old wisdom of the mind and body. As I will reveal in chapter 14, we even have instruments to communicate with long-dead survival entities, which may or may not fit the definition of being "ghosts".

It is time for medical practitioners to join the party.

CHAPTER 2

THE HISTORY OF ENERGY MEDICINE

The energy-based medicine paradigm has been a very long time in coming. In various forms it goes back to the depths of time and was (and still is) practised by shamans. The ancient Egyptians had a version of hands-on healing; the Ebers papyrus urges: 'Lay your hands on him to ease his pain and order his suffering to disappear.' It is entirely possible that the Bible stories of Jesus healing people recount a form of beneficial energy transfer.

HANDS-ON HEALING

Schiegl also describes the technique of *shunomatism*, named after a woman known as Abisag from Shuna who slept with King David to bring him back to health.[1] The concept of lying down with someone ill in order to take on their evil humours is told of in other tales as well. According to one story, Lady Bath of England slept with two young women; she recovered and they were left drained and ill. One might imagine other explanations for this type of recovery, but it is entirely consistent with Tantric teachings of energy transference.

PARACELSUS

The great Middle Age physician who called himself Paracelsus (Theophrastus Philippus Bombastus von Hohenheim) expostulated theories of health and disease based on an astral fluid, which we may liken to a bio-energy field and which he called *archea*. His method hypothesized sucking out the ill-humours or negative energy. He wrote about Earth magnetism, and readily spotted it had enormous power to influence our lives. In every way he was a visionary and brilliant man, centuries ahead of his time and someone who is still revered, and rightly so, by all practitioners of holistic and spiritually-oriented therapies. His major tract *De Origine Morborum Invisibilum* (*The Invisible Causes of Diseases*) nicely presages the title for my own present work! He would be pleased to see the revelations that science offers true-healing medicine described in this book.

ANTON MESMER

The other great figure who must be introduced in any review like this is Anton Mesmer. Born in 1734, he properly belongs to the modern scientific (post-Newton) age. Few figures have ever made such an impression on their era, or paid so dearly for assaulting the vagaries of medical orthodoxy. Even today his name is synonymous with smoke-and-mirrors mystification – to 'mesmerize' someone often means to somehow overthrow their common sense and harness their credulity. Yet this is to woefully misinterpret Mesmer's work.

Mesmer took some of his inspiration from earlier thinkers, including Paracelsus. He worked on energetic healing using systematic movements of the hands. Judging by the enormous numbers of people who came to him, he must have been very successful. He recognized a healing force of some kind coming through his hands; he even found he could transfer it indirectly through other individuals. He invented the term 'animal magnetism'. Unfortunately there was no way in his day to measure such a force field and he was ultimately discredited. Yet he was right, as we shall see. Today, just before the close of the 20th century, we are able to visualize the energies that he could sense and describe.

In Mesmer's work *Report on the Discovery of Animal Magnetism* he describes 27 axiomatic principles, which many enlightened doctors today would consider to remain valid. Only the terminology has changed. Here are a few of these key principles:

1 There is a mutual influence of celestial bodies, the Earth and human bodies [see 'the peculiar properties of water', page 110].
2 The medium for this influence is a universally present and continuous fluid, which permeates everywhere. It is

fine beyond comparison, and by its nature, is capable of receiving, spreading and communicating all influences of movement [the quantum field].

3 The mutual influence is subject to laws of mechanics that are as yet unknown [quantum mechanics].

4 The living body feels the alternative effects of this fluid: by penetrating the nerves, these are directly affected [neuro-peptide release; current model for much successful therapy].

Again, Mesmer was a man far ahead of his time and we have to move to the 20th century for further significant advances.

FIELDS OF LIFE

In the 1920s and 1930s Professor Harold Saxton Burr at Yale University began to experiment with electrical recordings of living energy fields of trees and, subsequently, humans. Trees were particularly suitable since they could be left wired up for long periods. Burr was fascinated to note changes brought about by sunlight and darkness, cycles of the moon, sunspots and seasonal changes.

Studying humans, he and his colleague Dr Leonard Ravitz noticed that human emotions affected this field. Voltages would be high when a patient was feeling good and would drop when he or she was below par. Burr foresaw the fascinating possibility that '... psychiatrists of the future will be able to measure the intensity of grief, anger or love electrically — as easily as we now measure temperature or noise-levels today. "Heartbreak", hate or love, in other words, may one day be measurable in millivolts.'[2]

Burr and colleagues also discovered a voltage rise just before ovulation, which drops just as the egg is released. Healing wounds also changed this voltage. Most remarkable of all, there were voltage changes due to malignant tissue and Burr was eventually able to predict, from reversal of the polarity across the abdominal wall, when a woman would in future develop cancer of the cervix.[3] This anticipates later prognostic work with electro-dermal screening described in Chapter 8.

What Burr and his colleagues were measuring was simply voltage potential. But he himself points out that changes can be measured at a distance from the affected organ or even outside the body, holding the electrodes above the skin, showing it is therefore a true field effect. He called it the 'Field of Life', or L-Field for short.

LAKHOVSKY

The next investigative genius was actually born in 1869; his seminal book *The Secret of Life* was published in 1925. This puts him ahead (chronologically) of Saxton Burr, but the reader will soon readily appreciate that progressively he belongs here in the sequence, since his visionary ideas look far forward into the world of modern bio-physics.

Georges Lakhovsky was a Russian engineer who became a naturalized French citizen and was ultimately awarded the Legion of Honour for his scientific technical services during the First World War. He had to flee his adopted country before the arrival of the Nazis, and died in New York in 1942.

Like those who went before him, Lakhovsky had to endure much calumny and ridicule. As one of his supporters remarked: 'The publication of *The Secret of Life* resulted in causing great annoyance to the custodians of infallible doctrines who made up with carping verbiage what they lacked in clarity of vision.'[4] As Lakhovsky himself put it: 'I have been attacked by physicists ignorant of biology and by biologists ignorant of physics who consequently can neither understand my theories nor judge my experiments.'[5] This extraordinary man of diverse talents showed that recorded sunspot activity parallelled magnetic disturbances and auroras on Earth. He also established a correlation between sunspot activity and good wine vintage years. In my own book *The Complete Guide to Food Allergy and Environmental Illness* I call attention to Lakhovsky's observation that geological terrain seems to have a potentially dangerous connection with cancer causation.[6] Clay soils in particular, he found, were dangerous, probably because of the properties of water within the soil, whereas sandy and limestone soils had a very much lower incidence of carcinogenisis. Lakhovsky also foresaw that one day it might be possible to project images of cancer tumours as an energy disturbance onto a TV screen; today we have MRI and CAT scanners.

But it is Lakhovsky's ideas about biological radiation fields that concern us here. His fundamental scientific principle was that *every living thing emits radiation*. This has important health implications. According to Lakhovsky, the nucleus of a living cell may be compared to an electrical oscillating circuit. This nucleus consists of tubular filaments, chromosomes and mitochondria, made of insulating membranes but filled by an electrically-conductive intra-cellular fluid. These filaments have capacitance and inductance properties and are therefore capable of working like radio transmitters and receivers.

> Some time ago, UK research scientist Roger Coghill extended Lakhovsky's insight by suggesting that the DNA molecule is the ideal shape (a spiral) for a radio-transmitting aerial. Perhaps the morphogenic field that tells an organism how to grow from its genes may in fact be an energy-message radioed from the DNA 'radio station'! (Coghill now considers it more likely to be the glyco-proteins – sugary molecules which stand up from the cell surface – which act like little aerials.)

In Lakhovsky's model, life and disease are a matter of a 'war of radiations' between the body's cells and microbes. If the radiations of the microbe win, disease and death will result. If the cell's own energy transmission wins, then health is preserved. Thus he arrived at a very advanced and quite defensible energetic view of disease. Lakhovsky himself went on to conduct very many experiments in this vein. The results he got were little short of startling for his time, and so one may presume there is a lot to be derived from his theories.

Albert Nodon, President of the Société Astronomique of Bordeaux, studying ultra-short waves in organisms, was able to prove Lakhovsky's hypothesis. He found radiation from all living plants and animals. Dead subjects did not, of course, transmit. Nodon produced remarkable figures showing that, weight for weight, radiation from certain beetles, flies and spiders was 3 to 15 times more intense than that from uranium. He extended his studies to humans and was able to show that our bodies emit even more intense energies than plants and animals. Nodon also obtained what were termed 'spontaneous radiographs' by placing living things directly onto photographic plates. Clear pictures were duly developed, after several hours exposure. This forgotten research anticipated Kirlian photography by many decades. Nodon's conclusion was 'It seems probable that matter, under the influence of radiation whose wavelength is less than the electron, may be subjected to certain modifications of an unknown nature which may confer new properties on matter, different from those conferred by radiations of a much greater wavelength, and not connected with electrons.'[7]

How right he was all those years ago.

For many years Lakhovsky had a great interest in the mechanism of cancer-formation. This in itself was unusual in his time. There were no 'Fight Cancer' media campaigns running then, and a leading London surgeon of the day pointed out that funding of cancer research did not even amount to one penny per person in the British Isles!

There have been many hypotheses advanced as to the causation of this pathological blight, including heredity, infection by viruses, local trauma, pollution and nutritional deficiency. It seems probable that all these factors may play a part. But Lakhovsky was convinced that oscillatory disequilibrium – that is, cellular radiation energy disturbance – was the predominant factor in the onset of malignancy.

The problem was, how to reverse it.

Our bodies consist of some 200,000,000,000,000,000,000 cells, and hardly any two oscillate exactly alike. This is partly due to differing tissues but also variation through time in the status of each individual cell. The impact of extraneous radiation would also produce modulations, such as the resonance effect. Finding a standardized harmonizing frequency would seem to be a Sisyphean task.

With brilliance and ingenuity, Lakhovsky invented his celebrated Multiple Wave Oscillator, generating a field in which every cell could find its own frequency and vibrate in resonance. The practical successes he began having in hospitals soon confirmed the validity of his theory. Numerous cases recovered and were documented by excited doctors.

Lakhovsky was careful to avoid talking in terms of a cancer 'cure'; however he did unequivocally cure a number of cases, and all the others showed variable but marked degrees of improvement.

If any reader would like to follow one of his simple experiments on plant cancer, it is not difficult to perform and will provide a fascinating home workshop on the properties of biological radiation. In this experiment Lakhovsky purposely dispensed with the oscillator and relied instead on the presence of ambient radiations. He took a series of Geranium plants inoculated with the Bacterium tumefaciens (= tumour-making) which causes

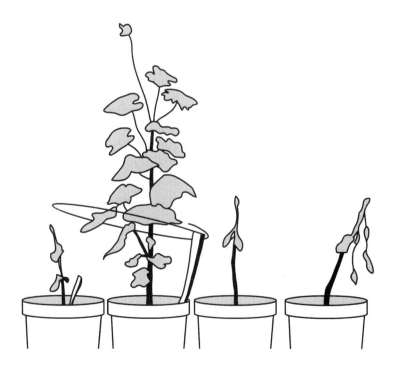

cancer-like growths on the plants:

> A month later, when the tumours had developed, I took one of the plants at random which I surrounded with a spiral consisting of copper and measuring 30 cm in diameter, its two extremities, not joined together, being fixed into an ebonite support [a rigid plastic tube, such as a spent biro pen stem, would suffice perfectly well]. An oscillator of this kind has a fundamental wavelength of about 2 metres (150 million Herz) and picks up the oscillating energy of innumerable radiations in the atmosphere.
>
> I then let the experiment follow its natural course during several weeks. After a fortnight, I examined my plants. I was astonished to find that all my geraniums or the stalks bearing the tumours were dead and dried up with the exception of the geranium surrounded by the copper spiral, which has since grown to twice the height of the untreated healthy plants.[8]

The oscillator was picking up and damping all kinds of atmospheric radiations. Lakhovsky bewailed the fact that so many radio transmitters were springing up (even in his day) that 'there is no detectable gap in the gamut of these waves'. Consider the health problem implied by this, when today we have a million times the intensity of blanket radiations that he experienced.

We will discuss this further in Chapter 10.

DR GEORGE CRILE

Famous US surgeon George Crile, founder of the celebrated Cleveland Clinic in Ohio, published almost contemporaneously with Lakhovsky, and their theories and predictions bear striking resemblances. I have chosen Lakhovsky mainly because, in my opinion, he was the more visionary of the two. Crile's radical work *The Phenomena of Life – A Radio-electric Interpretation* shows that he may be said to have discovered independently the same facts as Lakhovsky and used the same theories to explain his observation.

Addressing a congress of the American College of Surgeons in Chicago, October 1933, Crile pointed out that as the fundamental sciences of physics and chemistry advance their knowledge it should be possible in the future for the skilled radio-diagnostician to detect the presence of disease before it becomes apparent. If you want to know just how accurate this prediction is and cannot wait, turn to Chapter 8.

Crile foresaw Virtual Medicine.

THE SALAMANDER MAN

Enter Professor Robert Becker, orthopaedic surgeon and twice-Nobel Prize nominee. He is the first person on this list of pioneers and visionaries who is still alive today and making his views felt. He is noted especially for research into biological electrical potentials, but has gone on to become the doyen of energy medicine and the darling of the New Agers who, judging by fussings on the Internet, are looking for some scientific credence for their treasured mystical views.

However Becker is not to be much distracted by celebrity status and one can tell from his writings that he views being embraced by the alternative medicine movement with some alarm. He carefully distances himself from anything which doesn't fall into the strictest scientific rhetoric.

From years of experimental work on salamanders, showing that living organisms propagate a DC electrical field and that this undergoes certain changes when the salamanders are diseased and injured (exactly what Burr showed), Becker has developed elegant new theories regarding the electromagnetic regulation of life processes.[9] But Becker has gone further, with more advanced measuring systems, and has been able to show that body tissues act as semi-conductors, and that this is how the life-currents are transmitted. I find this exciting because it implies the possibility that living cells and tissues can function in the manner of a computer, providing there is suitable software (not that I think life is computer-modelled). So far, in my studies for this book I have not found anyone, not even Becker himself, who has had the same speculative thought.

Becker also showed, in his research into the subject of de-differentiation, that cells reverting to more primitive grades in response to stress (which is supposed to be impossible according to modern theories) not only takes place but can be deliberately provoked in frog red blood cells by a very tiny current which he measured in billionths of an ampere. Even a slightly stronger current did not have the desired effect, which would surprise the modern scientific community but not alternative practitioners, who have long understood the precept of gently coaxing a response from Nature rather than blasting it into action (which usually doesn't work). What Becker discovered is a version of the Arndt-Schulz low-dose homeopathic law given in full on page 120.

In the 1970s Becker and his biophysicist colleague, Maria Reichmanis, were funded by the US National Institutes of Health to study acupuncture scientifically. He chose to measure DC potential (electricity given off) at designated acupuncture points, and claims to have found that around 25 per cent of the points on the forearm were locatable using this method. He also showed that current is conducted by unknown channels which correspond to the stated acupuncture meridians. It is worth pointing out here that later in the book I will discuss research using changes in skin resistance at acupuncture points, which may be a more accurate method of detection. Proof of the probable nature of acupuncture meridians follows in Chapter 3.

Over the years Becker has expanded his authority and knowledge to be considered one of the best-informed scientists on the big issues of bio-physics and environmental hazards, particularly those concerning the effects of electric and magnetic fields on living systems. His recent book *Cross Currents: The Perils of Electropollution; The Promise of Electromedicine* is an extremely powerfully argued and comprehensive overview of what has been going on in the last two decades in the field of electro-biology. He didn't coin the term energy medicine, but he has certainly given it life breath and lifted it into the domain of science.

I particularly like his classification of energy medicine into three categories, according to the force used:

1 Minimal Energy Techniques: No actual physical energy transferred. Examples would include creative visualiza-

tion or hypnosis.

2 Energy-reinforcement Techniques: Adding to and supporting the body's natural energies. He cited acupuncture and homeopathy.

3 High-energy Transfer Techniques: supplying energy at higher-than-natural levels. Examples would be transcutaneous nerve stimulation (TENS), biomagnetics and electrotherapy.

This third category causes Becker a great deal of concern because of the biological hazards implicit in electrical and magnetic fields, the very subject of his book. He is almost a lone voice in pointing out the potential dangers of nuclear magnetic resonance imaging (MRI scans), so much the medical craze today. This investigative process subjects the body to huge magnetic fields and, as Becker explains, is probably not without theoretical risk, though this has never been properly addressed as an issue.

In the late 1960s Becker was probably the first person to predict that the magnetic field of the brain extends outside the head. He remembers how his idea was ridiculed by the audience at a scientific meeting of the time. Yet, he was eventually proved correct. This leads naturally to SQUIDs (without tentacles!)...

THANK YOU, MR JOSEPHSON

Finally today, we have gone on to develop instruments for the detection of biological energy fields. Notable among these is a device called the SQUID magnetometer. SQUID is an acronym for super-conducting quantum interference device. It is opening up a whole new world of bio-energetic science. The life field can be seen and mapped with an accuracy and sensitivity that would have been unthinkable 30 years ago.

The SQUID is based on a phenomenon known as the Josephson effect, after Brian Josephson, who predicted it in 1962 while working as a graduate student at the University of Cambridge. He received the 1973 Nobel Prize for his work. What his hypothesis means is that electrons, although we consider them particles (matter), can pass right through insulators as if they were waves.

Such a thing is impossible in the classical physics world, but natural enough in the quantum domain. We call this tunnelling and we now know that Nature has many examples of this, including events inside the human body!

A SQUID consists of a Josephson detector, with an array of input coils to capture the bio-magnetic field, plus the necessary electronics to amplify and make sense out of the signal thus received. The whole set-up is immersed in liquid helium which makes the device exceedingly sensitive to magnetic fields, such as the delicate ones given off by living tissues and organs.

MEASURING LIFE

What can we do with such a sensitive device? One of the first biological experiments with a SQUID was carried out by John Zimmerman, who developed the SQUID, and his colleague David Cohen at MIT's National Magnet Laboratory in Cambridge, Massachusetts, in 1970. They showed the heart's magnetic field with vivid clarity. In fact, it was still detectable 15 feet from the body.

Around the turn of the century, Dutch physician Willem Einthoven discovered electrical discharges from the heart. He received the Nobel Prize for Medicine in 1924 for this work. Nowadays routine electrocardiography is a standard part of the medical technological armoury.

Each heart beat is the result of an electrical discharge within the heart muscle; the current spreads to nearby tissues and can even be detected in the feet and hands. It travels in the blood which, being a salt solution, is an excellent conductor.

In 1821 Hans Christian Oersted showed that whenever an electric current flows in a conductor, a magnetic field is formed. If the current varies (*flux*) then the magnetism is even more intense. But the heart's magnetic field is very weak in ordinary terms, since the current is low. However, in 1963 Gerhard Baule and Richard McFee at the Electrical Engineering Department of Syracuse University, New York, used a pair of two million-turn coils (coils with one million loops of wire – that is, wrapped around the spindle one million times) on the chest of a subject and for the first time detected the heart's field.

It was in the same year that the tunnelling or Josephson effect was first published. Now SQUIDs can map the body's heart and other biological magnetic fields with amazing sensitivity. In 1971 Cohen went on to develop a brain magneto-gram or MEG (magneto-encephalogram). The brain's field proved to be hundreds of times weaker than the heart field, necessitating that the patient be electromagnetically shielded in the room where readings take place. Clothing must be free of any magnetic material, such as zippers, snaps and nails in shoes.

Since then there has been a real explosion in monitoring biological magnetic energy fields. It turns out that biomagnetic fields are often more indicative of events taking place within the body than are electrical measurements taken at the skin surface. For example, the eye acts as a remarkable battery and produces a substantial field which increases with the amount of light falling on the retina; we can obtain and study retinograms. Cohen himself, in 1980, reported detection of steady magnetic activity from growing hair follicles! Every muscle action creates a field effect

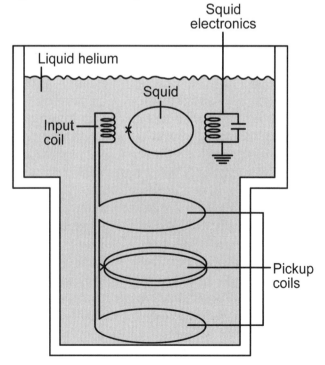

outside the body. SQUIDs even show that there is more intense cortical activity in finger control areas of the brains of musicians than non-performers.[10]

All this adds up to the fact that our living organisms are a field of teeming magnetic energy. There are other fields, too. These reflect what is going on within the body and, of course, it is entirely possible to influence the body in return. We live outside our skins! Life itself is an energy phenomenon. It no longer makes sense to practise medicine based on a biochemical or material paradigm; it's time to move over to the energy model.

So we can see that the magical, the mystical, the trendy and what was once dismissed as hocus-pocus in fact has a very sound theoretical basis in physics and can now be measured objectively, using the necessary scientific instruments.

RUPERT SHELDRAKE

We can conclude our list of thinkers by looking at the subject of information in biology. The view has long been held that all information needs some structural matter or energy system on which to be imprinted, otherwise it would have no existence in reality. It is now felt that information is somehow deeper than even energy systems; that information underpins physical reality and, especially, biological life systems. If this is the case, then energy is taking its orders from information fields.

In his book *A New Science of Life*, zoologist Rupert Sheldrake argues that all systems are regulated by something more than just matter and energy.[11] He hypothesizes that there are invisible organizing fields he calls morphogenic fields (morpho = form, genesis = making or giving birth to). These are informational fields, because they contain the detail needed to create the form, but they are not energy and therefore at this moment we cannot see them or make contact. We don't know how.

Since energy is not involved, neither are time and space. It follows therefore that the field does not attenuate with distance, as is the case with all forms of energy. It would also follow from these properties that fields can propagate effects across space and time in any direction, meaning past, present and future, here, there and everywhere at once. Actually, what Sheldrake is doing here is dressing up what we used to call 'magic' or 'supernatural' in the verbal metaphors of our age. It sounds plausible and therefore gets round resistance from die-hard thinkers. He can't prove his hypothesis, but it is attractive and self-sufficient; it covers many phenomena with no previous explanation. This theory has my vote.

According to Sheldrake's hypothesis, whenever one member of a species learns new behaviour, the causative field for the whole species changes. This would explain the famous '100 Monkeys' effect*. It also suggests that the dawning of the Age of Aquarius is more likely to be real than metaphor; that human consciousness is indeed going through some kind of collective evolutionary transformation.

Sheldrake's vision is hot stuff. He's a real scientific subversive, because it throws out Darwinian evolution and turns biology on its head. You can imagine the resistance to his theories based on the old scientific principle: *it can't be true, therefore it isn't*. If we had stuck to that one we would never have had vaccination, rockets, TV, anaesthetics, motorcars or heavier-than-air flight.

---

* **The "100 monkeys effect"** is widely misquoted and misunderstood. The term derives from a famous scientific study published in 1957, concerning a colony of the Japanese monkey *Macaca fuscata* on the isolated island of Koshima. One of the monkeys, a young female called *Imo*, taught herself to wash potatoes in a stream, before eating them. What astonished the researchers was not the intuitive genius of this particular monkey but the fact that once the proverbial "one hundred" monkeys had also learned to wash potatoes, within hours all the monkeys on that island, other islands and the nearby mainland all began to wash their potatoes before eating them. The conclusion is that once a kind of critical mass is reached, conscious awareness spreads by an analogue of telepathy. [Imanishi, "Social Behaviour in Japanese Monkeys", *Psychologia*, 1: 47- 54, 1957].

It was first introduced by Lyall Watson in his book "Lifetide"[12] and you should know it has since been hotly disputed that the scientists ever found such an effect (the sceptical tide!)

The fact is that thinkers ever since Darwin have been struck by the two snags in the plausibility of his theories:

1 There isn't enough time for the progress we see, supposing only the probability of Darwinian-style evolution.
2 There is nothing to say that new species were not created by some higher conscious control, even if 'natural selection' would subsequently favour their advancement. In other words, consciousness, implicate order or some other non-material force could be running the whole show and what we observe would be just the same. In short, Darwin's theory doesn't exactly fit the facts, but the idea of a creative, intelligent Cosmos with a guiding force that favours the life process over and above the mechanics of Newtonian physics certainly does.

Let's finish this chapter with the insights of Brian Josephson, Physics Nobel Laureate for 1973. He believes that the natural world is built upon a dualism of quantum mechanics and life force, analogous to the wave-particle dualism which vexed science for so long. The two together create what we ordinarily understand as "reality".

"The methods of the quantum physicist and of the biological sciences are seen to be two alternative approaches to the understanding of Nature, involving two distinct modes of description which can usefully supplement each other, and neither on its own contains the full story. The unified view explains the major features of quantum mechanics and suggests that biological systems may function more effectively than would be expected on the basis of quantum mechanics alone.

"Biology borrows results from physics and chemistry to obtain explanations for biological phenomena, thus explaining them with some degree of quantitative accuracy. Nevertheless, the fact remains that quantum mechanics is precision- oriented and biology process-oriented, and that to some extent the two goals are incompatible with each other".[13]

It's starting to sound like Eastern philosophy; let's go check it out!

CHAPTER 3

BIOLOGY BEYOND THE SKIN

One thing which the scientific scrutiny of biological energy is enabling us to do is re-evaluate older Oriental and other models of health, vitalism and body energetic properties. Often we find surprising concordance, and the realization is gradually dawning in the West that other models are not arcane or naïve constructs born out of ignorance but simply strange words attached to a very precise and more or less demonstrable and accurate body of knowledge.

This chapter proposes to visit some of these other energy-based models, the Chinese and Indian in particular. Each has aspects of which we will certainly need on our journey into the exciting world of Virtual Medicine.

THE CHINESE MODEL

Chinese philosophy, upon which Traditional Chinese Medicine (TCM) is naturally based, recognized an underlying ultimate reality which unifies everything. It was known as *Tao*, but this should not be confused with the later use of the same term by Confucius and his followers, meaning 'a path in life' or a code of conduct. In its original sense Tao means something very like our quantum field or zero-point energy; it is seen as something uniquely dynamic in character, flowing, ever-changing, creative and continuous. Thus the whole basis of TCM is energy and information; it is definitely *not* a substance-based medical model.

Tao also has the quality of being somewhat reflexive and circular – that is, coming back on itself, repeating endlessly rather than being linear. 'Returning is the motion of the Tao,' says the great classic *Tao Te Ching* by Lao Tzu, which also says 'Going far means returning'. This too reminds us of the new physics, which is teaching us a new reality that is flexible, flowing, reflexive and certainly non-linear. Effects become their own causes.

The well-known symbol the Tai-Ch'i T'u shows these several elements: change, movement, dark and light, circular, returning and complementary balance.

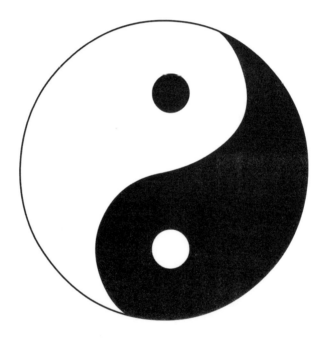

The two dots symbolize the fact that when one reaches the outer limit of a certain trend it must then reverse and come back on itself; each form or event contains the seeds of its own opposite. That's an awful lot of philosophy in one small motif!

Ancient Chinese medical theory is really a whole *gestalt* (composite) and it is somewhat artificial to separate out the parts. Life energy is called *Ch'i* and it flows in and around the body, constantly changing, interacting and influencing the physical domain. Blockages and disruption of the free flow of Ch'i is seen as the basis of disease. Other aspects of TCM include balance of energies (yin and yang), the five key elements (earth, air, water, wood and metal), the body clock (different organs dominant at different hours of the day) and the concept of Earth energies, or Feng Shui, interacting with all in a harmonious totality.

But what we are most concerned with here is acupuncture, the medical art of unblocking and balancing the flow of Ch'i energy through the meridians, or invisible energy channels, which run through and around the body. The practice of acupuncture goes back over 4,000 years, but its great flowering was the publication of a book called Huang Ti Nei Ching around 400 BC (The Yellow Emperor's Classic of Internal Medicine) available in translation by Ilza Veith [Berkeley, CA: University of California Press, 1993]. The use of fine metal needles, inserted at key points in the body in order to stimulate Ch'i, was evidently first introduced about this time also.

[Since first writing this I have spent time in Sri Lanka and seen evidence that acupuncture was present there long before the Chinese texts. For more information visit my website at:
www.alternative-doctor.com/specials/SLacupuncture.htm]

WHAT IS CH'I?

Ch'i is the word used to denote the vital breath or energy which pervades and animates all the cosmos. This sounds similar to the quantum information field or vacuum in which virtual particles come and go. Understanding the manifestation of Ch'i is central to TCM. It is also a key concept in which our Virtual Medicine theories come into direct contact with ancient wisdom, since there are remarkable parallels between descriptions of quantum probability fields and texts about Ch'i:

When the Ch'i condenses, its visibility becomes apparent so that these are then seen as shapes (of individual things). When it disperses, its visibility is no longer apparent and there are no shapes. At the time of its condensation, can one say otherwise than this is temporary? But at its time of dispersing, can one hastily say that it is then non-existent?[1]

This brilliant insight is quite remarkable. How could the author of this ancient text know that in centuries to come quantum physics would show that indeed the cosmos, far from being a vacuum containing fixed matter, would be seen instead as pervaded with information fields which cause 'matter' (virtual particles) to come and go as they need when interacting with something else? Again, our understanding of the true nature of disease turns on this point: if information energy of a disease is present but the disease not apparent, is it truly manifest? Or do we have to wait until structure alters and decays before we allow ourselves to be interested in healing? It is a crucial question, since now for the first time with Virtual Medicine we are able to see the forward projection of disease, before it becomes apparent.

In the human body Ch'i flows through discreet pathways called meridians and these affect the vitality and function of the organs. A blockage in a meridian will result in a malfunction of any organ through which it passes. It is worth pointing out here that a meridian passes through more than one organ and a disturbance in the meridian need not be confined to that organ alone. Thus for example the gallbladder meridian transects the canine tooth (eye tooth), upper and lower, as it passes across the face. An abscess in these teeth can cause gall-bladder dysfunction and vice versa.

Not only that, but we can bring in the 'organ clock' notion described in the Nei Ching. The gall-bladder meridian is dominant between 11 p.m. and 1 a.m. Thus the toothache is likely to be at its worst around midnight. Observations of this sort often astonish patients but are simple when you have the right medical model.

THE WINDS OF CHANGE
The meridians have been a source of great fascination to doctors and laymen alike in the West. Because of the craving for anatomical certainty, there has been a continued search to find some kind of structural explanation for the existence of meridians. They are clearly not nerve channels, blood vessels or any kind of duct system. Since no obvious anatomical struc-

tures mimic the described pathways of meridians, the tendency for Western science has been to dismiss the concept as something fanciful; this has not been helped by the choice of unusual metaphorical names given certain points such as *The Sea of Energy* (Conception Vessel 6), *The Marshes of the Wind* (Bladder 12) and *The Door of the Mental* (Heart 7).

Gradually the climate has changed. During the 1960s and 1970s the world's attention was increasingly drawn to Chinese traditions, partly accelerated by President Nixon's visit to mainland China. At around that time we first saw dramatic TV footage of major operations being carried out with no more anaesthetic than needles placed at exactly the right places in the skin. It was obvious to all and sundry that acupuncture worked, and worked at least as well as Western scientific medicine in some surprising ways, no matter how alien the rhetoric and however unfamiliar the mechanics and model. Since then, science has begun probing to see if it can establish at least some objective evidence for the Chinese model (evidence, that is, within its own paradigm and criteria of judgement).

We seem to have made a certain amount of progress.

THE NATURE OF MERIDIANS

In February 1937 the prestigious *British Medical Journal* carried an article by Sir Thomas Lewis describing a hitherto unknown network of cutaneous nerves.[2] He called it the 'nocifensor system' and deduced, from his experiments, that it was an independent cutaneous nerve system, unrelated to known pathways and unconnected to the autonomic nervous system. It was composed, not of nerve fibres, but a network of thin lines, similar to meridians.

In 1985 Pierre de Vernejoul at the University of Paris carried out a definitive and much-quoted experiment. He used a radioactive marker, technetium 99m, which he injected into subjects at classic acupuncture points. He then used gamma-camera imaging to track the subsequent movement of the isotope. He was able to show that the tracer migrated along the classic meridian lines, travelling quite quickly: a distance of

30 cm in 4–6 minutes.[3] As a control he made a number of random injections into the skin (*not* at acupuncture points) and also injected the tracer directly into veins and lymphatic channels. There was no significant migration of the tracer at other sites than an acupuncture point. What this simple but helpful study proved beyond doubt is that meridians are definitely real 'vessels' but they conform to no macroscopic anatomical structures whatever.

So if meridians are not nerve-conducting channels or other anatomically visible vessels, what are they? How is the energy conducted?

The answer is almost certainly via the collagen fibres of the connective tissues. As the name suggests, connective tissue fills in between the main organs and layers. There is thus a continuum of liquid crystalline water-bound collagen fibres running throughout the whole body. Recent studies have shown that these are not just mechanical fibres but that they have dielectric and conductive properties which make them sensitive to pressure, pH, local ionic composition and surrounding electromagnetic fields. In fact these collagen fibres, like a network mesh of fine electrical fibrils, form the ideal conductor medium in which many of the electro-magnetic phenomena described in this book may take place.

Even just disturbing and stressing these fibres gives off an electrical potential. You will notice when you have electro-acupuncture, as described in the Chapter 4, that the practitioner has the knack of 'massaging' the point he or she is testing, to wake it up and release this electrical potential in order to make a successful reading.

Remarkably, and very conveniently for us, this network of semi-conductor material can enforce a one-direction flow on the electrical current, acting rather like an electrical circuit with one-way gates called diodes. Once again, scientific testing has validated ancient wisdom and shown that the acupuncture meridians flow in one direction only – that which was described by the original *Nei Ching* text.

BODY CONSCIOUSNESS

The collagen network is of course in contact with the intracellular chemical fluid medium; this matrix in total provides an excitable continuum for rapid, coherent intercommunication throughout the whole living system of a human body. It is further the origin of the DC body field, as described by Saxton Burr and later Robert Becker (see Chapter 2).

This previously unknown dielectric domain could be described as a kind of body consciousness, separate from the brain and nerve cells, which is able to detect and retain experiences as a kind of memory, as well as register new experiences.

Interestingly, the fact that bound water plays an important role in consciousness was shown by evidence that anaesthesia may act by displacing bound water from membrane interfaces. Becker reported that general anaesthesia leads to a complete attenuation of the DC body field.[4] I have already remarked that acupuncture can render the conscious patient anaesthetized. Add this to the knowledge that some surgical patients feel pain even when (ostensibly) unconscious, and we can readily admit that brain and body consciousness are not the same and can be de-coupled one from the other.

THE AYURVEDIC MODEL

The ancient Ayurvedic healing tradition is considerably older than TCM, indeed is probably the oldest surviving model of health and disease. It has certainly stood the test of time and therefore deserves to be accorded respect. It would also prompt the wise scientist to begin asking what is workable about a system which has endured so long.

Once again, the zero-ground information field concept comes in: this time it is called *Brahman*, the ultimate reality. It is the soul or inner essence of everything and far transcends the ability to describe it in words (remember the difficulties of describing anything quite as weird as quantum physics). The word *maya* is used to describe how the ultimate reality of everything is made manifest in perceivable forms. It is often said that maya means the world is an illusion. Well, thanks to quantum mechanics we know this to be true at the subatomic level!

The universal energy, which the Chinese call Ch'i, is here known as *prana*. Instead of the meridians, the Indian system introduces the concept of *chakras*. These are the gates or channels by which the life-giving universal prana energy enters (and leaves) our bodies, thus influencing our bodily functions and vitality.

There are seven main chakras. Each one of these has a correspondence with anatomical structures, notably a nerve plexus and an endocrine gland. The name and correspondence of these main chakras is:

CHAKRA	NERVE PLEXUS	ENDOCRINE GLAND
Base	sacro-coccygeal	*gonads*
Sacral	sacral	*Leydig cells in gonads*
Solar plexus	solar plexus	*adrenals*
Heart	heart plexus	*thymus*
Throat	cervical ganglia	*thyroid*
Head	hypothalamus/pituitary	*pituitary*
Crown	cerebral cortex	*pineal*

What is less widely known is that texts refer also to other energy centres associated with major joint structures of the body, like the knees, ankles, elbows, etc. Taken altogether there are over 360 chakras of the body. These in turn are said to be joined together by a network of etheric channels called *nadis*, which are interwoven with the nervous system. Thus, unlike the TCM meridian system, chakras and nadis display considerable correspondence with anatomical structures.

Can we say anything about the chakras? What we need is hard evidence of their existence and significance. Unfortunately, this is singularly lacking. The best work to date seems to be that of Japanese psychic and clinical psychologist Hiroshi Motoyama. He is also a high priest and a yogi adept of some ability. At his research faculty, the Institute for Religious Psychology, he developed the AMI scanner, an acronym for Apparatus for Measuring

Chakra points

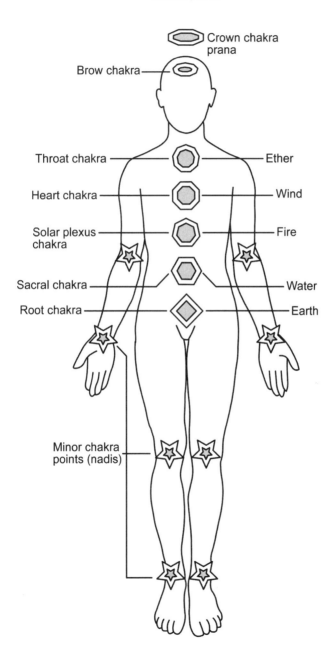

Crown chakra
prana

Brow chakra

Throat chakra — Ether

Heart chakra — Wind

Solar plexus
chakra — Fire

Sacral chakra — Water

Root chakra — Earth

Minor chakra
points (nadis)

the Functional Conditions of Meridians and their Corresponding Internal Organs (see Chapter 4).

Motoyama also claimed he had developed a 'Chakra Instrument' able to detect minute electrical, magnetic and optical variables in the immediate environment shell of the study subject.[5] The detectors have to be used in a light-proof room, shielded by lead sheeting on the walls and lined with foil which is grounded, to keep the electrical potential at zero. A 10 cm copper disc plus a photovoltaic cell (which generates electricity when light is detected) is positioned in front of the chakra being 'sensed', off the body. The magnetic detector is simply placed on the floor beside the subject – in other words within his or her magnetic field.

Changes in readings are processed and stored by a multichannel recorder, along with a number of conventional variables such as respiration rate, ECG and galvanic skin response (similar to a lie detector). Using questionnaires and evaluating disease susceptibility and organ function, and intercalating that with his 'detector' readings, Motoyama claims to have had some degree of success in objectifying the chakras. However the obvious criticism seems to be that he is depending heavily on the correlation between chakras and nerve plexuses. He could arguably be measuring nothing more than autonomic nerve activity, not energy vortexes in the ether!

SPIN

On the subject of vortices, this is probably a good opportunity to describe the phenomenon that practitioners using the systems described later in the book call 'spin'. In physics there is a phenomenon known as 'optical rotation', which comes from the helical structure of crystalline solids, or helical molecules in liquids and solutions. Spin is designated either right or left (dextro- or laevo-).

What practitioners with Virtual Medicine detector equipment have come up with is that healthy blood and saliva have a right-spin; urine and faeces have left-spin. When a person is under considerable duress or experiencing geopathic stress, this reverses.

Is it relevant? Certainly. Many patients with 'reverse spin' will not recover therapeutically until the spin is back to normal. The truth may be that spin-reversal makes one susceptible to outside events, such as geopathic stress, rather than vice versa.

But spin could have far wider implications. In 1995 I attended a conference in St Petersburg, in common with many other colleagues from the Scientific and Medical Network (a group of doctors and scientists dedicated to finding out more about the metaphysical and transcendent aspects of creation). There we heard lecture after lecture from leading Russian scientists about the properties of what are known as *torsion fields*.

Matter, we now know, has three basic physical properties: charge, mass and spin. Each of these gives rise to a characteristic field. Charge creates an electromagnetic field, mass gives rise to a gravitational field, and spin generates what we call a torsion field. It was high-level stuff, but what we learned is that torsion fields are different in having instantaneous effects at all points. Gravity fields have a distance effect, and electro-magnetic propagation has a time (frequency) effect, even though the ruling speed of light is pretty fast! Torsion fields, almost by definition, have neither a distance nor a time effect. In other words, we were hearing about a model which could explain telepathy and other supposedly etheric phenomena, which are so often dismissed as totally implausible.

I repeat once again my often-stated woe that if only doctors (and many other scientists) knew enough current physics, so much that seems strange and therefore improbable would yield to common sense enquiry. I was particularly pleased at the St Petersburg conference to hear through our discussions that thought could almost certainly be imprinted in space outside our skulls and left there for others to 'walk into'. There was a perfectly scientific explanation for certain strange and creepy feelings many of us experience from time to time. It could be the basis of déjà vu, though my Tunnels of Time project means I am heavily committed to the validity of past lives.

The potential for health effects from torsion fields, especially some of the strange outer-limit manifestations that you will read about in this text, is of course considerable. Readers will be able to work out many ways in which this obscure but enriching model could apply to the body-mind-spirit composite we call our Being.

WHAT ABOUT AURAS?

There is evident confusion about what is meant by an aura. Some consider it to be simply the energy shell around a person, which can become visible in certain circumstances. Others think it has metaphysical import. People claim to be able to see many layers of aura, which they attribute to the mental, emotional, astral and other aspects of the individual's composite being. I can only say that few can do this and therefore it is not truly objective. Further confusion is added by the fact that even I can see 'auras' around buildings, rocks and other formations, if the lighting and climatic conditions are right.

With this in mind, what objective evidence is there for such a thing as an aura? We will assume that it is identical with the L-Field or bio-plasma body mentioned in Chapter 2. There have been various attempts to make the total aura of a person visible. In 1911 Dr Walter Kilner, working at a London hospital, published a book entitled *The Human Atmosphere or the Aura Made Visible with the Aid of Chemical Screens*. He invented the Kilner screen, which was effectively a pair of glasses in which double screens held a liquid containing dicyanogen blue dissolved in alcohol.

Kilner described three zones around the body:

1 a thin dark layer close to the skin
2 a more vaporous layer, with rays pointing away from the skin
3 a tenuous outer layer about 6 inches across, with varying density and colours.

He found that this 'aura' would change with age, sex, mental energy and health factors. He was able to see shadows in the aura and could tentatively diagnose diseases such as hepatitis, cancer, appendicitis, epilepsy and psychological states.

Nowadays we can buy 'aura glasses' on the Internet. These are glasses with specially coated lenses which allow through only certain colours and screen out incident light. Some practice and concentration is required, but by all accounts most people can master it.

But the most definitive work to date in this field is the often-quoted study carried out by Dr Valerie Hunt and others at UCLA in 1977.[6] She had already discovered, using electromyography (EMG), that the body emits hitherto undetected oscillations between the 'noise' of normal muscle contractions. Using these as a marker she was studying the aura-energetic effects of a soft-tissue-manipulation healing technique called Rolfing (after Dr Ida P. Rolf, who 50 years ago called her work *structural integration*). To do this Hunt wired the subject to EMG electrodes positioned at the site of each major chakra, relayed to a recording booth where the sophisticated equipment monitored fluctuations in the electro-magnetic energy of the body.

But how to visualize the aura? Hunt brought in a trained psychic observer, Rosalyn Bruyere, who apparently could see human auras and the changes which took place in them. But was this really true? Hunt arranged to have Bruyere's descriptions and comments recorded synchronously with the changes in electro-magnetic measurements.

While the Rolfing therapy was taking place, Bruyere, who was obviously not allowed to see the physical recordings at this stage, reported changes in the colour and form of the energetic fields of the patient and Rolfer. Most satisfyingly, the patient and healer auras merged towards the end of the session as one identical shape and colour, something often described subjectively by hands-on energy healers and their patients.

The real test came when the recordings and aura descriptions were de-coded. It was found that changes in the patient's EMG status corresponded exactly with altered descriptions from Bruyere. Not only that, but when the frequency figures were subjected to mathematical analysis the Hertz bands suggested colours which also exactly corresponded with Bruyere's descriptions.

It is not too much to propose from this study that many energy healers get their results by superimposing a strong and reasonably balanced auric field (their own) onto the patient's disturbed and sick field; a version of shunomatism mentioned in Chapter 2. This isn't such an infringement as it sounds, since the two beings work together and seem to 'evolve' a new energetic unity that is somewhat bigger and beyond either one of them. This higher unity is able to heal and nurture.

MEASURING CHIGUNG

Most people today have heard of Tai Ch'i and its remarkable health benefits. Chigung is a more disciplined meditation, also using the power of Ch'i. Like acupuncture, this ancient practice is based on meridian theory. It is usually done sitting still with 'regulation' of breath (a relaxed concentration). Practitioners learn to monitor consciously the flow of Ch'i through meridians and channels in their bodies. Advanced practitioners can emit Ch'i with sufficient intensity that it can help others' ailing energies, forming the basis of yet another kind of energetic healing. There is also, evidently, an inhibiting Ch'i.

This ought to be detectable by scientific instruments. I have observed the beneficial effects on electro-dermal screening test methods discussed later in this book. But a more academic study was carried out by a group in the US and published in the *American Journal of Chinese Medicine* in 1991. Using infrared detectors, the researchers were able to measure output from the palms of advanced Chigung practitioners and concluded that at least part of the emitted Ch'i was in the infrared band of the electromagnetic spectrum. They were also able to show measurable levels of enhancing Ch'i emissions on human fibroblasts and boar (porcine) sperm. Facilitating Ch'i increased DNA synthesis, protein synthesis and cell growth in the human cells, while inhibiting Ch'i decreased all three. In the case of the boar sperm, different tests established that facilitating Ch'i increased respiration 12–13 per cent, while inhibiting Ch'i decreased it some 45–48 per cent.[7]

There no longer need be any doubt that science has crossed over into what was considered the etheric and is able to show a real effect. Of course measurements are made of electro-magnetic changes, not at the quantum level. But the body itself acts as the most sensitive quantum detector we have. Whatever is happening out there, it is real, not magic.

Now, surprisingly, we have machines which are actually capable of *generating Ch'i*. This is remarkable, because Ch'i masters have always felt that only living things could generate Ch'i. Even today, the only real detector of Ch'i is a sensitive and aware human being (a bio-detector). Dr Yuri Khronos, working with an Eastern-trained Ch'i master named Dong Chen, has been able to produce Ch'i electronically. Not only that, but it can be broadcast from tapes played through normal hi-fi loudspeaker units. Ch'i-aware people report rapid changes in their states of awareness from such broadcast recordings.

It is only a matter of time before Ch'i detectors are made. The impact of this on the development of consciousness is hard to foresee but will certainly be important (see Chapter 14).

PHOTOGRAPHS CANNOT LIE: OR CAN THEY?

In 1939 Semyon D. Kirlian, a Russian technician, was repairing hospital equipment when he noticed something strange. It was another case of the right mind prepared to benefit from a chance event; Kirlian thought it through properly and went on, with his wife, to develop what we now call Kirlian photography.

What he had discovered was that by the interaction of a very high-frequency electric discharge and a photographic plate, energy imprints of living organisms can be revealed on the film. The subject, enclosed in a light-tight bag, is in contact with a charged metal plate backed onto a photographic emulsion. At the moment of discharge, high-energy electrons jump from the plate to the subject, resulting in ionization of a thin layer of air between the two. The photographic emulsion is excited in the normal way and can be developed to reveal what may best be described as a visualization of the subject's energy field (which may or may not be the same as the aura).

Further research by scientists at the Kirov State University of Kazakhstan extended the discovery. They found that the light emanated was polarized (blue or red-yellow). This seems to accord with the traditional Chinese view of yin and yang energies.[8] These scientists began to refer to the visible energy shell beyond the body surface that was being recorded as *the bioplasmic body*. Studies showed it was affected by atmospheric conditions and cosmic events, such as sunspots. The Kirlians had already noticed rapid and pronounced changes in the energy photographed, caused by emotional disturbance. Increased light seemed to pour out with anger and (perhaps surprisingly) exhaustion. So here we seem to be looking at an actual visual confirmation of Burr's L-Fields (p. 19).

Experiments with plants and animals showed that each had a unique, defining energy field. What is most impressive is that even if half a leaf is cut away, the Kirlian photograph still shows the full field, the whole leaf energy appearing to be present even when the cut-away particles or mass is absent. Could it also be that the leaf 'ghost' photograph is defining one of Sheldrake's morphogenic fields? If not, what holds the energy vibration in place? It must surely be an information field of some kind.

The Kazakhstan workers also tried to record objectively the bio-physical changes that may take place in the hands of healers when treating a patient. What was visualized on the print when the hands of the healer were held close to a patient under the Kirlian camera was a narrow stream of energy, concentrating into an intense band which streamed into the area of the illness. What appeared to be happening was the transfer of energy from the bioplasmic body of the healer to that of the patient.[9]

Other applications of the photography, to demonstrate energetic transference of vital energy to water or seeds which had been held in the hands of a talented healer, were also successful. Photographs of manufactured or junk food show that it lacks the vital energy field which is present in and around fresh or whole food. The conclusion seems too obvious to comment upon.

In 1953 Dr M. K. Gaikin, a Leningrad surgeon, made an interesting discovery. He realized that the position of the main flares on the skin, which are characteristic of Kirlian photographs of humans, did not correspond to anything anatomical – but that they did appear at classical acupuncture points!

Naturally there has been hope that Kirlian photography will be able to offer the means to diagnose disease, based on imaging changes in the bioplasmic body. However, to date there seems considerable difficulty in distinguishing artefacts from true or meaningful photographic phenomena. Perhaps this may change in time. But for the present, few except the dedicated core of enthusiasts seem to take this remarkable technique very seriously. Thus Kirlian photography still has mainly the status of a party trick or an engaging exhibit at psychic fairs and carnivals, where practitioners charge a small fee for a 'picture of your aura'. Ironically, most of these aura-simulation cameras are not true Kirlians. There has to be direct contact with the plate, impossible at even a tiny distance or through a lens.

NOGIER'S SYSTEM

It is worth introducing here an odd offshoot of acupuncture theory called ear or auriculo-acupuncture. It was somewhat of a lost art but has been re-developed, particularly by French neurosurgeon Dr Paul Nogier. His system is based upon the image of a foetus projected onto the external ear and includes some 200 points. It has become widely adopted, even in China, where it has sparked a wave of research into the apparent embryonic connections.

Historically the Chinese, Arabs, Romanies, Hindus and some Europeans advocated needling a point on the ear lobe to remedy eye deficiencies. Even today some European doctors recommend the insertion of a gold or silver earring to stimulate this spot continuously in cases of eye deficiency. Currently auriculo-acupuncture is much used for anaesthesia, obesity and addictions such as smoking. An ancient Indian text, the *Suchi Veda* (which translated means 'Science of Needle Piercing') gives detailed techniques and points for needling the ears. It is interesting that the Arabs should use the ear mainly for the treatment of low

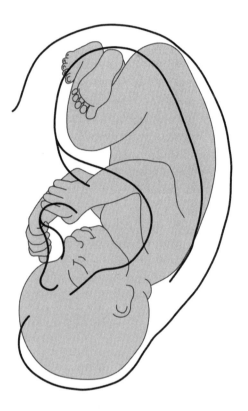

back pain and kidney trouble, when it is known that the ear is seen by the Chinese as the outward 'flowering' of the kidneys.[10]

The purpose is not to discuss the method here but to offset it somewhat against what was discussed earlier about the proving of meridians. If Nogier's theory is correct and there are connections from the ear points to each individual organ, we find ourselves very unsettled on the idea that meridians are anatomically proven. Indeed, it rather opens the debate up again. What had Nogier discovered? There is no arguing his powers of observation; many other people have confirmed the efficacy and accuracy of his correlations. But it does not rely on the concept of independent energy channels running through the body.

Rather, I think, Nogier's idea is one of neurological energy conduits projecting into the body field.

QUANTUM OPTICS!

Finally, I conclude this survey of biology outside the skin by calling attention to the theory of *ultra weak luminescence* or photon emission by living tissues, usually called "biophotons". This extends the work of Albert Nodon (p. 21), cited by Lakhovsky.

In fact biophotons were first postulated in 1923 by Russian medical scientist Professor Alexander G. Gurvitsch. He placed the roots of two onion shoots very close together and noted that they had a positive effect on each other's growth. If he separated them by means of a glass partition, this mutual synergy did not take place; however, if the dividing screen was made of quartz, the original mutual benefit was once again manifest. Gurwitsch concluded therefore that the growth influence had something to do with ultra-violet light emitted by the roots[11].

In 1974 German biophysicist Fritz-Albert Popp proved their existence, using sensitive photomultipliers, at the Max Planck Institute of Astronomy in Heidelberg. A case of progress having to await sufficiently sensitive instruments. What Popp showed was that clearer and more vigorous light emissions are associated with rapid growth, whereas this falls away with cell ageing. Perhaps most remarkable of all was the discovery that when an organism dies almost all its cells give up their 'death flash' at the same moment, some eight hours after the cessation of apparent life[12, 13, 14].

Actually, all objects, living or dead, emit a characteristic radiation, which is qualitatively and quantitatively related to temperature. This includes cells individually and the body as a whole. However, after compensating for these expected emanations, a significant number of photons (on the order of as many as 100 photons/cm_/sec) from living organisms have been detected over a range of wavelengths in the radio and microwave to ultraviolet range; this span includes radiation we are familiar with as light. The amount of light emitted is quite small; comparable to that observed from a candle viewed at a distance of 10 kilometres. Given the extremely small number of photons produced, for many years the predominant theory was that these photons were a random by-product of cellular metabolism.

In fact while science was underplaying the quantitative aspect, the qualitative nature of this light was being overlooked. It is phase coherent; that is to say, extremely highly organized. Given the random chaotic nature of the natural (physical) universe, it may be said that long range organization is peculiar to life (as I like to point out, it implies consciousness). Coherence is a defining quality of the biophotons. By its very nature, it has the power to hold information; information about living systems, enzymes, structures, dynamic processes, and, of course, disease!

Extending Popp's work, Herbert Fröhlich went on to study coherence and oscillations in biological systems. The fact that such oscillations are inherent in living systems means the resonance effect discovered by Abrams is based on solid science; indeed it is inevitable. As early as 1938 Fröhlich had became aware that a biological membrane supported an electrical field of 10 MV/m, which was way beyond synthetic materials of the time[15]. By 1974 Fröhlich had progressed to the point of showing that moist proteins behaved like moist ferro-electrics. Not only that but tissues had superconductance properties, even at room temperature. In physics this state could only be reached at temperatures just a little above absolute zero. Life was proving truly amazing.

Dr. Cyril Smith, from the Department of Electronic and Electrical Engineering of Salford University in the UK (who introduced a remarkable degree course in biomedical electronics) has gone further and avers that the living body is intrinsically a macroscopic quantum system and has adduced plenty of evidence for his hypothesis[16]. Essentially, that means we are a field phenomenon, extending to infinity, containing vast repositories of data, from past present and future, that define the organism as an integrated whole, interrelated as a system to all other aspects of the quantum field. This is what we may be talking about when we use terms like *Ch'i, prana* or the "Cosmic Web".

Now doesn't *Virtual Medicine* start to sound like religion?

It's time to put some of this fascinating background knowledge to work!

CHAPTER 4

THE BIRTH OF ELECTRO-ACUPUNCTURE

DR REINHOLD VOLL

Enter Dr Reinhold Voll, physician extraordinary. He is the very stuff of which legends are made: dark, irascible and arrogantly conscious of his genius. Originally trained in architecture, he qualified and became interested in technology as well as preventative medicine, an ideal combination to set the stage for his future. Voll contracted cancer of the bladder but refused to accept the Western dogma of terminal decline. Instead he sought relief through the intervention of traditional acupuncture methods. Remarkably, although he needed life-long catheterization, Voll conquered the disease sufficiently to continue working for over two decades – a testimony to the effectiveness of his teachings. Many people over the years have had cause to be grateful for this minor miracle.

Voll set about the business of trying to marry up Chinese medical wisdom with Western technology, a transition which had to come sooner or later, but with Voll it came soon, and comprehensively to boot. He began to survey acupuncture points and their related meridians, using a modification of a standard valve ohmmeter which he called the *diatherapuncteur*, and with it he founded the science of 'electro-acupuncture' in the 1950s. You may also at times hear of the *dermatron*, a later transistorized version of the same instrument.

The patient holds one electrode while the investigating physician uses a probe to complete the circuit by touching the skin at the point being tested. The small tip of the probe allows remarkable accuracy of placement, yet yields a great deal of information other than just skin resistance, as we shall see. The current is in the region of 10 – 12 microamps at a potential of 1.0 – 1.25 volts.

In other words, quite safe. Any more and the current itself would become stimulating and produce changes, instead of monitoring status quo. Indeed, just the very act of pressing firmly on the acupuncture point is sufficient to stimulate it, and very sensitive patients may even feel unwell due to this effect after such a test session.

Voll's first interesting discovery was that almost all Chinese acupuncture points are detectable by a change in skin resistance at that spot and are remarkably accurately located; most are within a millimetre or two of where the classic texts say. At these sites the skin resistance is a fairly constant 95,000 ohms (elsewhere the skin is highly insulating, at around 2 million ohms, except when wet). However, Voll also found many more such points than the *Nei Ching* and other classic texts tell us. So far this is simply a matter of scientific detection and there can be no argument; anyone who wants to measure these points for themselves can do so easily.

Additional Vessels

There are 12 main acupuncture meridians recognized in TCM and two principle governor vessels running in the midline, front and back (Conception Vessel and Governor Meridian, respectively).

It very quickly became obvious to Voll that there were other conducting channels, many extra points, and at least eight new 'vessels' were mapped, then labelled according to what he felt they represented in terms of biological function, namely: *lymphatic drainage*, *nervous system* (including the autonomic nervous system), *fatty degeneration* (including fat-soluble toxic chemical deposits), *organ decay* (including malignancy), *nonmalignant cystic fibrous and other benign degenerations*, *skin*, *joints* and *allergies*. His system brought the total up to 20 bi-lateral channels, two to each digit, fingers and toes, making a total of 40 channels in all.

There has also been the opportunity to rename some of the classic meridians with names more in line with modern Western science; thus the Chinese 'triple-warmer' has become linked with the endocrine system; the circulation-sex meridian (heart master) is now linked with vascular degeneration.

The illustration below shows the hands and feet and each vessel named on the Voll system. The only asymmetry is that the channel on the medial side of each big toe differs; on the left foot it is taken as indicative of *spleen* function, whereas on the right foot the same vessel is named for the *pancreas*.

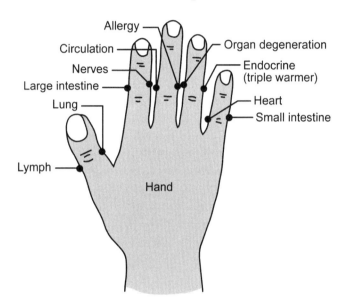

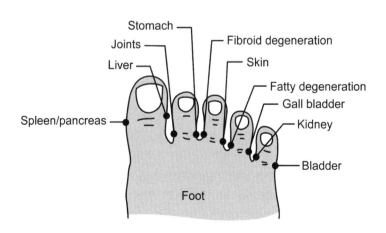

Too Much or Too Little Energy Flowing?

From here on it starts to become increasingly contentious. What Voll did is to arrange that a normal 'balanced' reading on a true acupuncture point is set at 50. At the upper end, 100, this would represent no resistance to current flow. A reading of 0 would mean total resistance (no current flowing whatever). Readings significantly higher than 50 on this scale mean too much energy (this may not at first sound an obvious problem, but remember all such excess energy must be stolen from somewhere else).

Generally we take readings of 65 or more to mean an excitation (or irritation). Over 80 is an active inflammatory process and over 90 an active inflammatory process that is pronounced in grade.

Conversely, readings below 50 mean degeneration and decay, which is more serious because destructive changes are less readily reversed. Below 40 is considered a sign of danger and below 30 an indication of an already established cancer or dead tissue (for example, I have observed readings as low as 27 at the point representing the defunct adrenal gland of a case of Addison's disease but without malignancy being present). I know of no EAV practitioner who has recorded less than 20 on this scale of values, but it would represent the final stages of tissue degeneration and death.

The scale of pathological readings is shown here schematically:

Value	Significance
90-100	Total '-itis'. Whole organ inflamed
80-89	Partial '-itis'
70-79	Cumulative irritations, premorbid
60-69	Physiological irritant values only
48-59	Normal range of variability
40-47	Incipient degeneration
30-39	Serious degeneration, pre-malignant
20-29	Advanced degeneration, almost certain malignancy
Under 20	Degeneration in the final stages

This may summed up as: *increasingly serious inflammatory and active organ disease above 80; serious degeneration and risk of malignancy below 40.*

Indicator Drop

In addition to the general level of readings, Voll recognized another phenomenon, which is where the reading is fine at first but after a few seconds it begins to die away to a lower level. What was *observed* is that the meridian somehow could not hold on to its energy. The *interpretation* of this is that there is disease tissue present somewhere in the indicated tissue of that meridian, influencing the energy levels.

Voll called this phenomenon the Indicator Drop (ID), and he considered this to be the most important reading of all. It points clearly to some significant pathological process taking place, regardless of what level the initial reading was found to measure. Put another way, a meridian which is high but where there is no Indicator Drop is not nearly so much a problem as one which reads nearer 50 but has a major drop. For example, a high liver reading (90+) means a major detoxification is going on, with high liver energy and possible inflammation of liver tissue. Voll called this reading the 'speeded Indicator Drop' and declared it indicative of chemical intoxication. But providing there is no die-off effect, the problem lies elsewhere. The liver overburdening is a secondary manifestation. The source of the toxins is the matter which needs rectifying, which when solved will ease the liver problem.

Basically, the bigger the Indicator Drop, the more serious the pathology giving rise to it. The electro-acupuncture practitioner will seek out the biggest drop in the measurement system and choose to treat that first, as a priority. This leads almost inevitably to the concept of 'most stressed organ' and implies a necessary treatment regimen.

Correlations

Where Voll became decidedly controversial is the systematic way he went about trying to find correlations between each electro-acupuncture points and specific organs and diseases. In my view he may have been stretching his cloth to fit!

Most scholars of the Chinese system are content to view the 'gall bladder' or 'large intestine' meridians as concepts or qualities of energetic potential, rather than being related necessarily to disease of those organs. Voll thought otherwise and, over many years of painstaking and detailed research on many thousands of clinical cases, he gradually catalogued enough data to be able to associate certain points with certain organs or relevant tissues.

Gone was the old system of colourful metaphors such as *The Sea of Energy* (Conception Vessel 6) and *The Door of the Mental* (Heart 7). Instead, in Voll's system, the first point on the endocrine meridian is associated with gonadal and adrenal function; the fifth point on the heart meridian connects with the mitral valve (left) or tricuspid valve (right); the ninth point on the lung meridian is larynx, and so on (all examples counted from the tip of the relevant digit, whether the start or finish of the meridian).

Existing meridians were found to have several additional points, so a new naming system had to be devised. The first point between 1 and 2 became 1a. Then came a 1b. But then further divisions led to 1-1 and 1-2 and so on. The result is confusing but there is a certain amount of consistency based on function. For example, Voll considered the second Voll-point on each finger (just distal to the last knuckle joint) to be concerned with lymphatic drainage, so these are always designated 1-1; the point immediately proximal to the last knuckle joint he associated with the sympathetic plexus of the system concerned, and these are always designated 1a. Conveniently, Voll's method concentrates mainly on taking readings on the hands and feet and nearby skin, so the patient is spared much disrobing.

Eventually Voll published a complete knowledge system of all the above which we now call 'electro-acupuncture according to Voll', or *EAV* for short. It is the first real model outside Abrams' original work of what I have chosen to call *Virtual Medicine*.

Criticism

As a user of the EAV method with some years' study it is possible to say that there are indeed some remarkable correlations between EAV points and meridians, but overall, I feel that Voll has invited criticism by trying to fit the clinical findings into his mental hypothesis. After doing so he has come up with a useful but partly inaccurate 'map'. That said, there is nothing that even comes close in scientific terms to such an advanced energy diagnostic system and it does indeed go a long way to combining the intuitive genius of the Chinese system with the preciseness of Western electronic technology.

Perhaps, as the idolization accorded to Voll fades into a brilliant historical perspective, it will be open to others to question some of the master's dogma and make changes which reflect more accuracy in what is being tested and more humility concerning the fallibility of the method.

Central Measurement Points (CMPs)

There are many points to measure, over a thousand in all. We don't try to measure every one on each patient. An obvious question would be: is there any way to establish quickly the general state of each meridian? One suggestion is to measure the ends of the meridians. These points are called 'Ting points' in Chinese nomenclature.

Without going into the arguments for and against, it has been settled that it is better to measure a little further up the meridian, at what we call the central measurement point or CMP. With one or two exceptions, like the thumbs, big toes and heart meridian (inside of the little finger), this point is just distal to the second knuckle joint. This gives an overall idea of the energy of that meridian. If there is suspicion of a problem then it is very simple to delve deeper and check other points related to that meridian.

By using the CMPs as quick reference points it is usually possible to home in on the problem area. However, nothing in EAV overrides the common sense of history taking. If the patient says she has lung problems and the CMP has no Indicator Drop (ID), it is mandatory to check other points on the lung meridian.

As with conventional medicine, electro-acupuncture is about establishing a hypothesis as to the causation of illness and then dealing with it. The fact that different criteria and an unfamiliar frame of reference are called into play does not alter this basic logic or mean that we ignore what clues there may be in the patient's description of his or her problem.

PRACTICAL CONSIDERATIONS OF EAV

EAV is not easy, though simple enough in concept. It is rumoured that it takes five years to make a good EAV specialist. That may be true, but being able to get useful readings and helpful therapy pointers can be learned in a matter of days. After all, one does not need to be a brain surgeon to learn to dress wounds and set up an intravenous line. Consistency of probe pressure is the hard part to master. Once the practitioner can do that, everything else follows.

The real difficulty is to learn the remedies. It's a whole different repertory (see Chapter 7) and certainly does take years to get to grips with. But there are always textbooks to help.

It is also important to respect certain general rules. We know, for instance, that testing after a heavy meal obscures the results. We call this a *parasympathetic dominant state*, when the patient is lethargic and the energetic system somewhat closed down (yin state). But TCM tells us more: that, as in all things, the body cycles through contrasting phases; midnight to noon is a time of sympathetic dominance (yang); noon to midnight is parasympathetic dominance (yin). Moral: don't test after about 6 p.m. and never after the patient has eaten a big meal! These are things one learns gradually.

Other factors which can reduce a patient's energy are lack of sleep, severe stress, cold or medications.

Quadrant measurement

A quick and easy test to see if the patient's energies are adequate for EAV testing is what we call *quadrant measurement*. It can be shortened to a hand-to-hand reading. Provided the energies fall in the 80–90 range, there is sufficient energy for testing. If not, some means of stimulating the patient is required. This could be having the patient run on the spot, clap his or her hands together forcefully a few times, or tap repeatedly on both temples.

Quadrant testing is a useful preliminary procedure. Readings are taken from hand-to-hand, right hand to right foot, left hand to left foot, and foot-to-foot (foot measurements are made with the patient's soles on electrode plates). If there is a significantly higher or lower reading in one of the quadrants compared to the other three, it suggests that the key pathology is in that quarter.

Hypothalamic Disorder

Sam Williams, Jr, an advanced EAV specialist physician, taught me the importance of checking hypothalamic status. It happens sometimes that when recording meridian energies at the CMPs that everything seems 'irritable' – that is, a great many small Indicator Drops register, but nothing really stands out. This makes it difficult to know where to enter the case. Systemic steroid therapy can produce a similar picture, where IDs are being clearly suppressed. However, in this case there is usually some reading which enables us to break into the problem.

Screening for hypothalamic disorder is done by measuring at the traditional Chinese point of Triple Warmer (TW) 20, which lies just above the ear pinna. Measurement is made while the patient is in contact with the ground with one hand, touching TW 20 with the probe.

Alternatively, the patient uses the index finger of the hand holding the bar electrode to touch TW 20, while the therapist uses the probe on the allergy vessel CMP of the opposite side. An imbalance of readings on the two sides indicates either hypothalamus disorder, or possibly a dislocation of cervical vertebrae at the level of C3 or C4.

If one or the other condition exists, it will skew the results and it would be best to remedy this problem first. Subluxation will need a realignment manipulation by a skilled chiropractor or osteopath. If it is indeed a hypothalamus problem, matters can be improved by choosing a suitable restorative remedy or light therapy (see Chapter 9).

Unless a hypothalamus offset is corrected first, the therapy regime will not be totally accurate and consequently less effective.

Foci

Using electro-acupuncture, one is given several new insights into the disease process that are not obvious to the traditionally-orientated clinician. For example we have the concept of a 'focus' (plural: *foci*). No matter what the presentation of the patient's complaint, it often emerges that there is some area of the body which is distressed and 'transmitting' a trouble signal which influences the energy body adversely.

Common examples would be old tonsillitis, appendicitis, what I call pelvic 'anger' in a woman, prostatitis in a man or teeth and gum problems (see Chapter 12 for startling new revelations about the dangers of teeth foci). These foci can appear 'silent' clinically but they are certainly not so electromagnetically.

When a focus is active within an organ tissue it will disturb the body's homeostatic regulatory mechanism. The body needs to divert a great deal of its energies to cover up and compensate for the focal disturbance. This causes imbalances in other organs, with fatigue and global low energy states. Therapy may be blocked until the focus is corrected.

It soon becomes evident to the budding EAV specialist that these hidden and smouldering foci are quite dangerous and can create a great deal of chronic ill-health, rather like the 'smouldering virus' that we began to talk about in the 1960s. Spread of infection and toxins by blood transportation is obvious. But another largely unsuspected route is retrograde seepage along nerve channels. We know that viruses and bacteria *can* travel in nerves: rabies, herpes and poliomyelitis are just three diseases where this is known to happen. In 1923 two groups in Paris and the US chanced upon identical experiments. Each inoculated rabbits in the eye with Herpes simplex virus ('cold sore' virus) and showed clearly that the virus tracked along the trigeminal nerve to the brain stem. This is the critical area of the brain pathways, where all the key functions converge. What wasn't said, though quite obvious and pointed out by Patrick Stortebecker of Sweden (of whom more in Chapter 12), is that teeth are also supplied by the trigeminal nerve and dental foci could also track into the cranium and attack central brain tissue in this way.

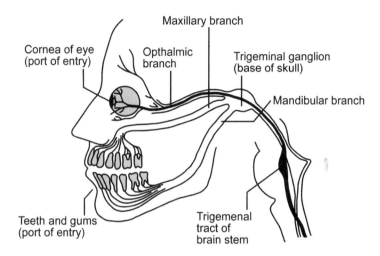

Payling Wright, pathologist at Guy's Hospital in the 1950s, showed the poliomyelitis virus and even inert substances such as ink particles and dyes could travel at a remarkable 2—3 millimetres an hour (5–7 centimetres a day) in this way.[1] Unfortunately, this kind of observation is not given any currency and the vast majority of doctors and medical students do not know of this phenomenon and the appalling health risk it poses.

REMEDY EVALUATION

If the testing system described so far were not enough for a lifetime of work by one man, Voll gave us another gift of technological insight. We call it 'remedy evaluation'. How this came about is ascribed to one of those lucky accidents, a case of the prepared mind being ready at the right place at the right time to be able to benefit from what, to others, would merely be a baffling observation.

Let Voll tell his own story:

I diagnosed one colleague as having chronic prostatitis and

advised him to take a homeopathic preparation called Echinacea 4X. He replied that he had this medication in his office and went to get it. When he returned with the bottle of Echinacea in his hand, I tested the prostate point again and made the discovery that the point reading which was previously up to 90 had decreased to 64, which was an enormous improvement in the prostate value. I had the colleague put the bottle aside and the previous measurement returned. After holding the medication in his hand the measurement value went down to 64 again, and this pattern repeated itself as often as desired.[2]

Voll went on to verify this startling discovery with many other patients and found it to be consistent and very helpful in choosing appropriate treatments.

Thus was remedy evaluation born, though Abrams and Boyd had reported it earlier (Chapter 1) and it was subsequently forgotten.

How It Works

Part of the EAV circuit includes a test plate or a 'honeycomb' – that is, a metal block with slots to take small phials of test substances for comparison. The plate has to be on the passive electrode side of the circuit, so that the remedy 'signal' has passed through the plate and *then* the patient, before being picked up by the probe and completing the loop back to the instrument (See illustration opposite).

If we accept the presence of the Indicator Drop as indicative of a pathological process somewhere along the meridian system, then logically any remedy which removes that drop and restores the reading level will have a beneficial impact. We can put a remedy into the circuit and test the response. If it improves matters somewhat but does not eliminate the adverse read completely, it is open to the practitioner to add other likely therapeutic agents until a satisfactory formula is obtained. Thus we can build a therapeutic regimen with the assurance that it is at least *likely* to work.

Dr Kuo-Gen Chen of the Department of Physics at Soochow University in Taipei has researched medicine testing extensively and explains that 'When a medicine sample is put on the metal plate of the EDS (electro-dermal screening) circuit, the electron waves passing through the plate will be phase modulated. When these waves later pass through the patient's body, a given signal is transported to the proper organ or tissue by resonant absorp-

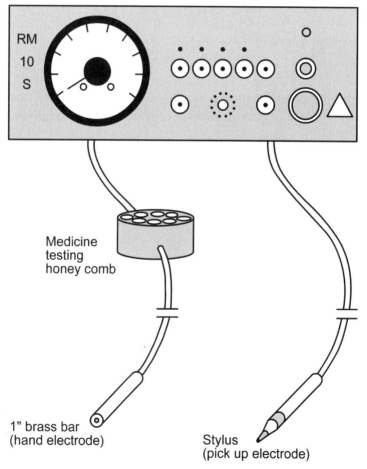

Test meter (12 microampere)

Medicine testing honey comb

1" brass bar (hand electrode)

Stylus (pick up electrode)

tion.' In his view, testing is an application of *quantum mechanical quasi phase matching.*[3]

Rapid large-scale testing of remedies can be done by arranging racks of trays containing large numbers of phials. The Dermatron or other sensing device is then connected to each rack in turn; when a rack reads positive, individual trays are tested until the right one is identified; finally each individual phial in this tray can be switched into the circuit until the necessary remedy is located.

In this day and age you would expect computers could help and you would be right. We come to this in Chapter 8.

ALLERGY TESTING

The alert reader will probably quickly deduce the reverse side of this remedy-testing coin: *that it is possible to identify substances which bring about an Indicator Drop where there previously wasn't one and therefore assess them as harmful.* If bringing milk into the picture produces the same Indicator Drop as weedkiller, the therapeutic implications are obvious.

Thus one of the applications of EAV is to look electronically for 'allergies'. After more than two decades of work in the allergy field I can add my own comment here. I have many times observed that patients can become ill without ingesting or breathing their allergens. Sometimes just close proximity to the reagent can do it. In 1987 a young woman from Hong Kong flew over to see me in the UK. Her problem sounded bizarre; but she told it to the right person, because I believed her. Karen Rackham said she felt ill if she was merely in the same room as a cup of tea! It was indeed an allergy and subsequently we were able to help.

Providing the substance comes into the individual's L-Field, it can cause energy disturbance (remember the L-Field extends to infinity but in practice falls away very quickly, according to the inverse square law). Thus there have been many occasions when a highly-sensitive patient has had to be moved to the other side of the test room, away from the racks of testing substances.

I am now convinced that allergy is primarily an information field effect and not a biochemical or humoral one. The neutralizing solutions or vaccines of the Miller method, described in full in my earlier books, are simply another energy medicine dispensation and this explains why putting the neutralizing dose under the person's tongue sometimes works almost instantly. The relief can occur before there is any time for a humoral transfer via the circulatory system. This clinical observation accords very well with the theories of Professor Jacques Benveniste, who holds that all molecules have an electromagnetic information signature which itself can produce the same clinical effect as the molecular substance, even when no chemical is present. He likens it to listening to Pavarotti or Elton John on CD, when the artiste is not actually present.[4]

Naturally, this is highly controversial and regarded as little more than quackery by many doctors. But if one accepts the validity of the Indicator Drop and what it is telling us, this application of electronic allergy testing is at least consistent with the rest of the EAV system.

Is There Any Supportive Proof?

Naturally any scientifically-orientated doctor would want to see some objective proof of what EAV can do. I am pleased therefore on two counts to report two small-scale studies by Julia J. Tsuei and others using EAV to evaluate food allergies and hypertension.

Tsuei received her medical education in China, Taiwan and the US and naturally has a strong affinity for TCM; acupuncture in particular. She has been engaged in several research programmes to further the scientific credibility of acupuncture and Voll's electro-dermal technique.

The food allergy test was simple but sound. Thirty volunteers were used. Allergies identified by the Voll method described above were compared with findings from five other recognized allergy tests: history, skin tests, RAST, IgE levels, and food challenge testing. Voll testing correlated well, particularly with results from challenge tests which, logically at any rate, should tell us the most about food allergy (personally I have strong reservations about the use of food challenge tests as the benchmark in scientific trials).[5]

Tsuei and her team carried out another study on hypertensive patients which is also worth reporting. There were 336 participants, 171 normals and 165 hypertensive individuals. Measurement points were selected based on either TCM or Voll's hypothesized correlations, totalling 56 points tested on each participant.

The 56 points could be divided into seven groups, of which two were measuring cardiovascular energy, three were not, and a further two groups measured both cardio-vascular and non-cardiovascular points. The first group, measuring only cardiovascular energy, correlated extremely well with systolic and diastolic blood pressure, and the other cardio-vascular group also correlated with left-ventricular mass (hypertrophy due to excess blood pressure). Indicator Drops (IDs) on these points gave the most accurate method of identifying the hypertensive patients. But there were also significant relationships between IDs and left-ventricular mass and either systolic or diastolic pressures among three of the five remaining groups.[6]

THE MECHANICS OF EAV

Voll's work was furthered by Professor William A. Tiller of the Department of Material Sciences and Engineering at Stanford University in California. During the 1970s Tiller and other material scientists were investigating the properties of skin to determine the requirements for prosthetic skin, which could be used to treat burns and other skin graft procedures. They studied elasticity, resistance, permeability, chemistry and many other biological properties of skin.

Some researchers, including Tiller, were surprised to find that certain points on the skin had much lower resistance than elsewhere. They knew nothing of Voll's work but soon realized that what they had located were acupuncture points. Tiller studied the dynamics of acupuncture points. The data obtained during these investigations revealed a complex, changing system of information. His model grew to include several electrical properties, such as resistance, conductance and capacitance:

Conductance is the reverse of resistance and measures how well electrons flow.

Capacitance is caused when charge builds up across an electrically resistant barrier; there are several such layers in the skin.

All of this means that skin conductivity is far more subtle than just the properties of a wire cable. Many factors play a part, the cells of the different skin layers influencing the diffusion and permeability of electrically-charged ions such as sodium, potassium and chloride ions. Tiller began to refer to acupuncture points as 'windows of information'. According to his model, the health status of the organ in question affects the concentration and diffusion of ions at the points along the meridian, and thus the rate of electron flow, which is what EAV measures.

We need far more studies in this area. Unfortunately, research in the alternative medical field is grossly underfunded. We are lucky, therefore, when an academic institution chances to become interested in this way.

CAUTION

It is very important for the reader or potential patient submitting to EAV to remember one thing, which is that what we are measuring with this system is energetic disturbance. It is *not* equivalent to a blood test or special x-ray, demonstrating gross pathology. We can find the energy signal of cancer of the colon and yet *absolutely nothing can be detectable clinically*. The energetic system is saying that trouble may be coming and be able to characterize what the likely nature of it will be. Obviously there is great preventative potential here. But there are strictly no grounds for disputatious exchanges with conventional doctors or accusations of 'missing' the diagnosis.

This sometimes poses great difficulties for EAV practitioner (many of whom, it must be said, are *not* qualified doctors anyway). A natural desire is present to try to persuade conventional physicians to investigate what has been found energetically and see if there is confirmatory structural or biochemical evidence of disease. But one is inviting ridicule and hostility by revealing one's source of the diagnostic suspicion. Perhaps it is not conceited to hope that the publication of this book will prove helpful when these ticklish situations arise; it could be given to the uninformed physician as a primer.

Casebook: Female, 38 Years

Stan Richardson, a capable if medically-unqualified Voll practitioner in Heckmondwicke, Yorkshire has the following remarkable story to tell:

A woman telephoned one day, asking for help, saying she was sick and frightened she would die. Could Stan help?

When she attended, she looked ghastly and even Stan was concerned. Without allowing her to explain anything, he sat her down and surveyed the initial points. It showed serious drops on the stomach, small intestine and large intestine meridians. Only *then* did he ask her, 'What's been happening?'

She explained that for over three weeks she had been suffering from overwhelming diarrhoea and vomiting. She could keep nothing down. Medicine from the family practitioner was ineffective. She had lost over 3 stone (40 lb) in weight and was frightened but preferred to see an EAV specialist she trusted, rather than attend a hospital.

Stan then resumed and stopped, quite puzzled, when he found a strong resonance that said *rabies* was present in the stressed organs. He didn't tell the patient this but asked the quite reasonable question: 'Have you been abroad lately?' The patient answered that she had just come back from India and been ill ever since she'd arrived home.

'Were you bitten by any animal?' Stan asked; again a very pertinent question. The woman insisted that she had not. Eventually, Stan had to reveal to the patient that the signal from her tissues was rabies. After discussion it emerged that this woman, in her misguided kindness, had been feeding dogs with kitchen scraps at the back door of her hotel in Delhi each night. Clearly what had happened is that she had been licked by a rabid animal and had swallowed the virus from her own fingers, resulting in the appalling intestinal symptoms.

Normally, rabies is spread by a bite which breaks the skin, the virus enters the nerves and travels backwards to the brain, where it is deadly. She had escaped a fatal disease by amazing good luck.

Stan supplied her with a mixture of homeopathic medicines which remedy-testing had said would be beneficial. Her symptoms ceased within 24 hours. By the end of the week she had gained back 10 pounds and eventually made a rapid and full recovery. She had fought, and won, a serious medical battle within her body, using nothing more than quantum energies.

The importance of this illustrative Virtual Medicine story is not merely that it is dramatic and life-saving. It is that *no conventional doctor in his or her right mind would have diagnosed rabies in this situation, or even considered it*. Yet the virtual energy signal showed quite clearly it was present, and with a suitable remedy led the patient back to safety.

Otherwise, she might well have died of severe 'gastro-enteritis', without the hospital doctors ever suspecting what the cause was.

MOTOYAMA AND THE AMI

It would be neglectful to write a chapter describing Voll's work in favourable terms without at least mentioning a similar and contemporaneous development by Tokyo clinical psychologist (also priest, yogi and psychic) Hiroshi Motoyama. His 'Chakra Instrument' has already been discussed on page 40.

Motoyama's AMI system (*Apparatus* for Measuring the Functional Conditions of *Meridians* and their Corresponding *Internal* Organs) is based on the principles of TCM. It was designed to detect organ excess or deficiency by measuring the response to a 3-volt electrical stimulus, sampled at very high frequency. It calculates four different parameters from which the diagnosis is made:

1 autonomic nervous system
2 flow of Ch'i
3 immune system
4 organism's response.

Measurements are taken on the Ting points (end points of meridians) using a double-layer electrode which is totally free of pressure artefacts, unlike Voll's data collection. The clinical information derived is useful, and arguably this system is the most reliable and objective electro-dermal diagnostic test.

Dr Julian Kenyon of the Centre for the Study of Complementary Therapies in Southampton, UK, has carried out a statistical analysis of three machines: the AMI, the segmental electrogram (SEG), from the Vega stable (see Chapter 5) and Kirlian photography. Kenyon dismisses Kirlian photography as worthless, with a co-efficient of variation of over 50 per cent; his own system, the SEG, was 35 per cent and needed to be under 15 per cent ideally. But the AMI returned accuracy at the level of 5–10 per cent (different for each of the above four parameters but all within this excellent range). According to Kenyon, this 'Puts the AMI in a class of its own when compared to other electrodermal diagnostic devices'.[7] What may eventually prove more significant is that the AMI has now been adopted by the Japanese government for official medical screening technology, which is a most satisfactory step forward in Virtual Medicine.

This device is definitely a milestone and is odd, in that it is a Western energy medicine device from an Eastern source!

CHAPTER 5

THE VEGATEST

It is said that Reinhold Voll submitted the last few additions to the EAV system a matter of days before his death. Whether this is whimsy or truth, it is clear that he achieved remarkable things despite the blight of a terminal illness. His life work completed, there was little point in going on suffering.

Two subsequent, related developments emerged during the 1970s. Both came into clinical use while Voll was still alive. We shall look at each in some detail in the next two chapters.

The basic problem with Voll's raw method was that it was complex and difficult to organize the data gleaned in a meaningful hierarchical manner. Many points had to be tested and he was gathering *too much* data. It was thus a very laborious and time-consuming procedure which made it exhausting for both the patient and the practitioner.

Starting in the early 1970s Helmut Schimmel hit upon a simple improvement which was to stay with only one testing reference point, usually on the hand for convenience, and introduce diagnostic test ampoules containing low-dose homeopathic extracts of different mammalian organs (usually pig). Applying the same logic to the meaning of an Indicator Drop, if the pathological reading appeared when the liver D4 ampoule was placed in the circuit this would infer problems with the patient's own liver. The test organ ampoule was energetically resonating with the distressed organ tissues within the body. Schimmel called his instrument the Vegetative Test Machine, or Vegatest for short (often just 'Vega').

Again, the core diagnostic indicator is the drop in energy (decrease in measured skin resistance), coupled with a musically falling electronic wail. As with all EAV devices, I find that practitioners tend to test 'by ear', not just by needle deflection. Schimmel named this cadence the *'disorder control'* and it is calibrated at the start of testing by introducing some poison into the 'honeycomb' of the EAV circuit (the test plate – a metal block with slots to take small phials of test substances for comparison – see diagram page 65), such as an ampoule of Paraquat or Lignocaine. It is not easy to master the use of this indicator, but those who can manage it have at their disposal a rapid and approximately accurate means of testing large numbers of organs, pathogens and likely treatments.

PRELIMINARIES

Vega testing is measuring extremely fine energy oscillations, either in the quantum realm or connected with spin phenomena described on page 42, or some unknown mechanism. This makes it highly susceptible to 'noise' and corruption of signals. Proper observance of start-up procedure is therefore important.

The test room must be free from geopathic stress (see page 170). Computers, x-ray machines and other electronic apparatus should be situated well away from the test zone (or at least switched off), making certain there is no interference from equipment in adjacent rooms or even above and below the test room. Electromagnetic fields travel through walls. Even electrical cables give off a substantial magnetic field, and for normal household and commercial voltages the patient must be seated at least 70 cm (2 feet 4 inches) from the nearest power source and at least 1.5 metres (5 feet) from any fluorescent lighting.

It is important that the tester is not personally geopathically stressed, otherwise he or she is likely to 'find' this condition on all patients. In fact if any condition keeps arising in consecutive cases, the first thing the astute BER (bio-energetic resonance) practitioners think of is that they are picking up their own disorder.

The practitioner needs to be in good shape health-wise, and well-rested. Sick patients are often in a predominantly yin phase and tend to drain the practitioner's energies (even lay-people may notice this effect with certain invalids). An exhausted tester cannot get good results. You may notice that the practitioner wears a peculiar magnetic belt. This is said to provide additional protection when testing. Nevertheless, it is unlikely that the practitioner can realistically test for more than a few hours per day without becoming substantially yin and unable to get meaningful results.

CHOOSING THE REFERENCE POINT

Just as in EAV, the Vega specialist tests on an acupuncture point. The tips of the fingers are readily accessible and are chosen by preference: the so-called 'Ting points' just at the corner of the nail bed. The allergy vessel, endocrine or connective tissue meridians are common preferences.

A point has no testing potential unless it can first be made to give off a disorder read, so the practitioner begins by establishing this important pre-requisite. Gentle probing should give a reading around 100 and when a poison is introduced into the metal honeycomb the subsequent reading drops markedly. Ideally, the fall should be 20–30 points on the scale. If this is impossible to obtain, then amplifiers are introduced, in this case ampoules of Epiphysis D30 (30X), until the reading is sufficient to be useful (the homeopathic dilution scale is explained in Chapter 7). The amplifiers are left in the honeycomb throughout the testing session.

Obviously, since the same point is being used over and over, it may well become traumatized and cease to give off any further disorder control. This is especially liable with a beginner using nervous, heavy-handed pressure. Another point has to be selected, but it must be checked for a disorder read before proceeding.

STRESSING THE BODY

It may seem surprising at first, but the body often needs stressing lightly in order to unmask energy disorders. The body's own bio-energetic compensatory mechanisms can be remarkably good at covering up a problem (a reason why normal medical diagnostic skills may be needed as well as an interest in these new methods).

Under normal circumstances the body will always endeavour to obtain a homeostatic balance of the energy flow within the body and the surrounding field. Sometimes only when an additional burden is imposed on the body do masked disturbances become noticeable. Ideally, we would like to choose a mild stressor that produces no harm and is soon re-balanced after testing.

In practice the best approach has been found to be a small electrical shock applied to Lymph 1 and Allergy 1 (points suggested by Voll). A piezo-electric device called a PM 2000 is generally used, which administers a mild charge of 4,000 volts per millisecond. It sounds scary but the current is mild and the patient rarely feels anything at all. Alternatively, the Vega machine also has a 13 Hz provocation output which can by used. This is a stressor frequency (low beta).

The body is thus required to make a compensatory response, which will divert the masking energies and expose real pathological readings which could otherwise be missed.

FINDING THE STRESSED ORGANS
As quickly as possible the Vega tester wants to get to grips with the most stressed organs. This is where the key pathology lies and where the therapeutic response is going to be maximum. This is done by testing a series of organ ampoules, usually at the D4 (4X) potency.

Testing can be speeded up by testing brackets or racks of test ampoules simultaneously. A bar connected by a wire to the honeycomb and laid across several ampoules at once gives a result which is referenced to all those ampoules. If a read appears, then one of the ampoules is active. This can be located by examining them one by one. If the whole bracket is negative, then all of them can be set aside and time has been saved.

The knowledgeable Vega tester will learn to relate what shows up to the patient's clinical condition. It is of course possible that he or she is unaware of any relevant subjective symptoms. Let me once again repeat that the search is for an energetically disturbed organ, which will not necessarily be 'diseased' by the criteria of Western laboratory medicine. We correct the disturbance, Nature does the rest. Only if the energy is left untreated may pathology ensue.

FILTERS

The range and sophistication of the Vega machine is greatly extended by the use of what Schimmel called 'filters', that is, extra ampoules of test reagents introduced into the circuit which modify the response. Reagents have been chosen empirically, and supposedly give further information about organ status and the disease process. For example, here is a list of filters and what they tell us about a disturbed organ:

Zincum met D400	Severe organ stress
Zincum met D200	Most stressed organ
Zincum met D60	Critical organ stress
PhosphorousD32	Most damaged organ
Ars. Alba D60	This is the origin of the patient's complaint

I have already introduced the concept of a focus in the previous chapter. Filtering with the homeopathic remedy Thuja D30 will show a focus is present, and this can be related to the relevant organ. Causticum D60 shows a focus with a disturbance field. There is actually a certain logic to these potencies; thus Causticum D400 (more potent) shows a *dominant* focus with a disturbance field. Generally, the higher the potency that reacts, the more severe the disease.

If the clinical condition is caused by or associated with psychological disorder, a number of emotional filters can clarify matters further. Thalamus D4 will show a neurological disturbance based on autonomic dysfunction. Epiphysis D4 tells us that psychogenic stress is present. Mandragora radice D30 shows exogenous depression, and at the D60 potency tells us it is endogenous in nature. Hypothalamus D800 shows psychosomatic illness; Epiphysis D400 shows hypersensitivity.

Geopathic stress has become a matter of keen interest among alternative practitioners. Chapter 10 investigates aspects of this issue is detail. Meanwhile, the Vega system claims to have filters which can tell us more about a patient's problem:

Geopathic Stress Filters

Silica D60	Geopathic stress present
Iron filings	Geomagnetic stress
Quartz sand	Curry grid
Cuprum met. D800	Double grid stress
Phosphorous D60	Electromagnetic field stress
Agate	Yin stress (discharging field)
Calc. carb. D1	Yang stress (charging field)
Radium bromide D1000	Ionizing radiation exposure
Silica D2000	Frequency stress

Other filters can tell us if the patient is yin- or yang-dominant (linseed oil and sugar water, respectively), mercury toxic (Merc sol. 30), vitamin-deficient (Manganum D200), enzyme-deficient (Zincum met. D200) or hormone-deficient (Molybdenum met. D200).

I have some problem with the nature and efficacy of these 'filters'. They were largely developed by Schimmel and seem very subjective, as well as empirical. However, I do accept that the Staufen pharmacy, which prepares the ampoules, manufactures strictly ethical products, using dilutions of real-time substances to create the filters.

Something is going on, that is clear; I know a case where Radium bromide D1000 read on a woman patient – it emerged her husband worked in the Sellafield Nuclear Power Station. The tester knew nothing of this at the time. Did she carry minute traces of radioactive material? If not, what strange quantum ripple or 'etheric' message was picked up by the woman from her spouse and carried to the practitioner's clinic?

I find these matters fascinating and filled with the richness and luxurious mystery of Nature, rather than an affront to my scientific training. I just think it is high time that proper evaluation studies were carried out and we got past the 'empirical' stage which has now dragged on until one could call it entrenched opinion.

The Vega machine manufacturers are fond of attacking other people's technology. It is time they applied the rules to themselves. What little material is published is mainly in German and this does not advance the international stature of this potentially enlightening test system.

STRESS INDEX

A novel and useful concept, introduced by Dr Erwin Schramm with his Neo Bio-Electronic Test, is that of 'biological age'. It was taken up by Schimmel and also appears in a number of subsequent devices (see page 197). This has nothing to do with calendar age (years) of the test patient but with the vitality and resistance of his or her tissues. The higher the biological age, the more prone the body is to decay and malignant processes. A more descriptive term might be 'stress index'.

Schimmel used potentized embryonic mesenchyme tissue as the reference test agent and gave a range arbitrarily calibrated from 1 to 21. A filter of Cuprum met. D400 is put into the honeycomb. Apart from amplifiers this is the only ampoule used, and it will set the 'disorder control' (see page 74). One by one, starting with 21 and working down, the Mesenchyme ampoules are put in to test; if the Vega reading reverts to 100 (the reference point or pre-requisite of Vega testing, indicating no disorder) this is positive.

Usually testing shows a high age (representing the pathology), a mid-range value (representing the body's present resistance capability) and a low value which is felt to be the 'optimum' biological age for that person.

Reference ranges are shown here:

1–6   These represent the range of normal cellular respiration and do not normally need treatment.

7–10   Indicate pre-clinical phases or functional disturbance with clinically manifest changes.

11–13 Usually clinically recognizable disease.

14–15 The beginning of chronic degenerative changes. Pre-malignant.

16–17 Possible micro-malignancies may be present.

18–21 Possible macro-malignancies which need to be tracked down.

Readings above 10 are usually a sign of clinically manifest disease.

The idea with therapy is to help the patient get down to his or her 'optimum biological age' value. But those who teach the Vega method explain that it is unwise to try to come down to the optimum age too quickly, otherwise unmanageable homeostatic stresses, which decrease the body's ability to recover rather than enhance it, may appear. Gradual improvement may take several sessions and a number of different remedies to drive out the disease signal and attain a suitable biological age.

REMEDY FILTERS
The Vega system obviously includes the capability of remedy testing, along the same lines as Voll's method. Possible remedies will give harmonious balanced readings; unsuitable remedies will create or increase the disorder control.

In fact we can be more refined in this. A number of filters introduced into the honeycomb *prior* to remedy testing will increase the success rate markedly. Thus, for example, filtering with the ampoule Ferrum metallicum D800 will eject remedies which are not going to be *tolerated* by the patient; Ferrum metallicum D26 shows it will be *effective*; and Manganum metallicum D26 shows it will be *compatible* with other remedies selected.

Homeopathic remedies, as you will read in Chapter 7, can sometimes have strong effects on the patient, even when ultimately beneficial. It is important to avoid causing too much unnecessary disturbance, since this rarely assists the true course of healing. This triple bracket of remedy filters is helpful in getting the balance just right.

ORGAN THERAPIES
Voll and Schimmel have given us the concept of 'the most stressed organ' and this has naturally led to new therapeutic regimes. Why treat a pain in the foot if the precipitating cause lies in the liver or adrenals? Obviously, medication to enhance organ function is the logical path. Unfortunately, there is the stigma of patent medicines attached to such an approach (I still remember my mother's 'Little Liver Pills'). The fact is that centuries of herbal lore and specialist healing knowledge go into these compound

formulas, which is more than can be said for most of the allopathic medicine range, where treatments come and go like fashions as they are found to be too toxic and then swept under the carpet. The truth remains that there are considerable degrees of lowered function before gross pathology finally appears. It is right to give the body support at *this* stage, not when pathology has finally engulfed the organ. This is so elementary, one wonders why the medical profession has such a struggle with the simple logic involved. Conventional tests for liver function require alterations in blood status or actual anatomical structure before a diagnosis of disease can be made. Yet these changes represent the final *failure* of the body to compensate. Long before that stage, Nature is working hard to keep everything going as it should, a nip here, a tuck there and a little bit of patch and mend. This is hardly optimal, and yet doctors will so often pronounce 'Your blood work is normal, *therefore there is nothing wrong*', when manifestly there *is* a problem and the patient feels unwell. It can be a question of degree.

Here is where energy medicine triumphs because it measures the electrical status of the organ and monitors its function as a whole. One might think of an 'organ gestalt' (whole composite). Subtle changes in this complete electrical field can reflect the fact the several different functions aren't working exactly as they should, while yet there is nothing majorly wrong.

Organ support could include a vitamin and mineral panel, such as my adrenal stress formula, digestive enzyme aids (to boost pancreatic insufficiency) or a liver nutrition formula. This can be combined with physical measures such as a coffee enema to stimulate the liver (common procedure with cancer cases), or colon cleanse where parasites and other bowel toxins are suspected.

SIMPLE LIVER CLEANSE

If you are not getting any results on therapy after three weeks; if you had an initial good result but have started feeling unwell again; or if you have had many years of toxic build-up (drugs, alcohol, tobacco, etc.), you may benefit from a detox programme and a simple liver cleanse.

If you have started a detox programme, this may release further toxins from the fatty and connective tissue where they have been lurking. Sometimes body metabolism can't cope properly at these times and you may go into an overload crisis. Typical signs would include:

- feeling heavily hung-over in the morning, even when you've not been drinking
- slow getting started in the morning
- feeling unduly tired or drained
- having a very low tolerance of alcohol.

There is no need to attempt the extremely heroic 'liver flushes' sometimes in vogue in the alternative field. There are claims that you will release showers of gallstone gravel but this is nonsense. What actually happens is that you pass granules or pellets of saponified olive oil, which you are supposed to swallow in huge amounts (a litre at a time) in these misguided procedures. It's a hoax, basically. The give-away clue is that these "stones" float in the toilet pan. Only fat is lighter than water!

Instead try this simple formula for 10 days (you can then repeat it a few days each month):

Recipe
- 6 tablespoons of lemon juice
- 3 tablespoons of virgin olive oil (cold pressed)
- 1 small garlic clove, crushed
- Pinch of grated ginger
- Pinch of cayenne pepper

Whisk in a blender and drink immediately. Do not eat for at least 1 hour afterwards.

The acid test, of course, is treating the energetically ailing organ and being able to observe the resultant recovery in health. Whereas no method of testing and treatment is foolproof, the Vegatest approach gives successes often enough to be considered a very valuable attack on the disease process.

PHENOLIC TESTING

A special and very useful application of the Vegatest is that of phenolic testing. I have written about this in my previous book *The Complete Guide to Food Allergy and Environmental Illness.*

In 1979 Dr Robert Gardiner, Professor of Animal Science at Brigham Young University, Utah, began to speculate that his own allergies might be caused by a sensitivity to certain aromatic phenol-based compounds that are found naturally in plant foods and pollens. He acquired some of the pure compounds, made serial dilutions and began to experiment by taking sub-lingual (under the tongue) doses and noting the results.

Sure enough, he found that some phenolic substances reproduced his main symptoms. Not only that, but neutralizing these reactions with subsequent low-dose antidotes of the Miller-method type effectively solved his allergy problems. He was able to eat most foods without reactions. He experienced a major improvement in health.

In other words, allergy to coffee might really be an allergy to chlorogenic acid which is found in the coffee bean. Injecting the chemical produces the same allergic wheal and flare response as the food itself would. There are many such compounds in food. Milk contains 13, tomato has 14, soya 9. A little expertise in these phenol families leads to new allergy diagnostic skills. For example, someone reacting to beef, milk, banana, yeast, potato and tomato might actually be allergic to nicotinic acid. The table overleaf gives a number of common foods and their phenolic content.

PHENOLIC COMPOUNDS IN SOME COMMON FOODS[1]

Compound	Found in
Apiol	almonds, beef, carrot, celery, cheese, milk, oranges, peas, rice, soya beans
Capsaicin	milk, onion, potato, tomato
Cinnamic acid	apple, banana, beet sugar, celery, cheese, grapes, lettuce, milk, onion, oranges, peas, tomato
Coumarin	apple, banana, beef, cane sugar, carrot, celery, cheese, chicken, egg, lamb, lettuce, oranges, peas, potato, rice, soya beans, tomato, wheat, yeast
Eugenol	almonds, beef, carrot, celery, cheese, milk, oranges, peas, soya beans, tomato
Gallic acid	almonds, apple, beet sugar, cabbage, cane sugar, carrot, celery, cheese, egg, grapes, lettuce, milk, onion, oranges, peas, potato, tomato, wheat
Malvin	apple, cabbage, carrot, celery, chicken, egg, grapes, lamb, lettuce, milk, onion, soya beans, tomato
Menadione	apple, celery, egg, grapes, lettuce, onion, peas
Nicotine	beef, milk, potato, tomato, yeast
Phenyl isothiocyanate	beef, cabbage, chicken, egg, lamb, milk, onion, peas, soya beans, tomato
Phlorizin or phloridzin	apple, beef, beet sugar, cheese, egg, grapes, lamb, lettuce, milk, orange, soya bean, yeast
Piperine	beef, beet sugar, cheese, chicken, grapes, lamb, milk, onion, peas, potato, soya beans, tomato, yeast

Piperonal	almond, beef, beet sugar, cabbage, lamb, lettuce, milk, tomato, yeast
Rutin (quercitin)	apple, beef, beet sugar, cane sugar, carrot, celery, cheese, chicken, egg, grapes, lamb, lettuce, milk, orange, pea, potato, rice, soya beans, tomato, wheat, yeast
Vanillylamine	almonds, apple, beef, cheese, grapes, lamb, lettuce, milk, onion, orange, potato, soya beans, tomato, yeast

The story was taken up by Dr Abram Ber, who began testing patients for sensitivity of this type with a Dermatron. He was able to claim success with a wide diversity of complaints, particularly in infants and children, getting excellent results with autism, dyslexia, insomnia, enuresis, respiratory allergies, abdominal pains and asthma. In adults, remissions were achieved with many chronic problems such as migraine, fatigue, depression, asthma, arthritis, colitis, hypertension, menstrual problems, skin diseases, chronic constipation and cardiac arrhythmias.

People struggling against their allergies suddenly found a whole new dimension of management for their condition. This can rightly be ascribed as a major benefit of the Vegatest system, or any EAV derivative. Intradermal testing of these compounds would be slow, painful and time-consuming. The Vegatest is quicker, non-invasive and far cheaper to administer than hours of intradermal tests, though as someone who has done both I believe it is not as accurate and is subject to the cautions discussed in the following section on objectivity ('Considerations', below).

Some phenolic compounds have been found to correlate well with certain diseases. Cinnamic acid (in fruits, cheese and nuts) is a major cause of skin irritation in eczema and other dermatological conditions; coumarin (wheat, rice, barley, corn, soya, cheese, beef and eggs) contributes significantly to arthritis; malvin (found in some 35 common foods, including chicken, egg, corn, milk and soya bean) may be associated with autism, dyslexia, learning difficulties, epilepsy and other neurological disorders in children.

There are many other phenol-based compounds which are crucial to our physiology, such as neurotransmitters (serotonin is one), hormones, co-enzymes and pharmacological food ingredients such as caffeine, enzyme inhibitors and anti-nutrients.

The Vegatest is used to establish neutralizing dilutions in just the same manner that any remedy testing is carried out. The ideal antidote would be that which eliminates the disorder read when an allergy filter is in the honeycomb. The patient takes these neutralizing dilutions sub-lingually for a month and then returns for re-testing. The aim is to get down to the first dilution (5X), meaning that the patient has become fairly tolerant of the allergen. He or she can then use a weekly or twice-weekly maintenance dose.

CONSIDERATIONS

The Psychokinetic Effect

Vega testing requires more skill than EAV but both are difficult to perform well. The clumsy Vega probe is certainly part of the problem. I myself learned to use this technique in the 1980s and it would not be right to withhold from the reader that the machine tends to give the practitioner what he or she expects. In other words, I liken it to 'electronic dowsing'. Those who watched Schimmel himself at work observed that he often varied his probe pressure and seemed to know what he was going to 'discover' before he found it.

This raises the question that the disorder control (or indeed Voll's Indicator Drop for that matter) are no more than subconscious muscle responses to a preconceived mental intuition. In a world of supposed objective science, this standard of testing may seem a little strange; it may not sit comfortably for some. Therefore it is vital to make clear to the reader that any such 'objectivity' is a myth. No scientific study has ever been devised which eliminates the element of operator intrusion. This is one of the main things that quantum physics has taught us.

This is a widespread problem in energy medicine and subjective practitioner "detection" techniques. I feel I need to warn the reader that many would-be health investigators are deluded. Dr. Hulda Reger Clark (not a medical doctor) published a book entitled *"The Cure for All Cancers"*[2]. In it she describes tests in which she, the operator, "diagnoses" cancer in the patient and then, a week or two later, announces to the happy patient that he or she has been "cured". Even the most liberal alternative practitioner could not and should not accept this shabby standard of science.

That's not to say she is wrong in proposing organisms and substances have unique identification signatures. That's the whole premise of the Virtual Medicine model (see chapter 13 for more).

But this good lady seems unable to understand that if she has a fixation that all cancers are caused by the parasite *Fasciolopsis buski* and iso-propyl alcohol, then that is what she will find when she "tests" for them. That doesn't make it true!

It is not supporting evidence to point out that many patients get well with her treatment. Many patients get well anyway. Nor is it enough to say more patient get well than with conventional anti-cancer therapy; because the population she deals with is highly motivated towards alternative survival and self-help. Many of these will fight their way to a recovery, with or without her ideas.

If Dr. Clark gets positive results at all (and I'm told she does), then I wager it is because of the adjuncts to her theories, namely that patients are encouraged to de-pollute, eat a good diet and take adequate nutritional supplements. There is ample proof that this helps the fight against cancer; so it does not mean her ideas hold water.

In the same way, practitioners who are constantly finding the same thing on their patients should try to be honest in self-appraisal and ask the question whether or not they are finding their own story all the time. This can mean pet obsessions and narrow thinking; or it could mean that the practitioner in question has the disease personally and is misinterpreting the findings to mean it is a signal from the patient!

Naturally, you may expect that this teaching isn't popular with would-be practitioners. But I can only tell it as I see it and encourage you to be cautious in evaluating the truth.

In fairness, leading Vegatest practitioner Dr Julian Kenyon acknowledges the inevitable inclusion of the psychokinetic effect and defends it heavily. As he says, 'It is important to recognize the part played by the practitioner in bio-energetic regulatory techniques such as the Vegatest method. This does not detract from their validity but merely means that the Vegatest and similar methods are looked at for what they are, no more and no less. They are however easier to carry out than using a totally psychic effect such as in dowsing because an objective subtle electrical change is taking place.'[3]

Dutch worker Van Wijk investigated this further in 1989.[4] He carried out studies on EAV performance. Voll's method of point testing was addressed in great detail and it was found that a pressure of 125 grammes was optimum. At this level the variability of resistance was less than 5 per cent. The average recovery rate of refractory skin tissue at this optimum pressure was 10 seconds. Van Wijk really showed that changes in conductivity are pressure-sensitive and independent of electrical current which, on the face of it, undermines Voll's work.

However, in 1992 Van Wijk showed that trained practitioners could identify an 'active' ampoule among 19 blanks over 90 per cent of the time (1:20 probability).[5] This is a far higher rate than chance and considerably better than conventional medicine recovery rates.

The Human Detector

My own view is that the human organism is capable of operating as a sensitive quantum bio-magnetic detector and that the results are at least in a degree objective. In other words the tests can be blind and the operator will sense something; that 'something' will lead to a subconscious alteration in probe pressure. I judge this valid scientifically. However, a great deal more investigative work needs to be done, otherwise all this is food for the critics. It does not serve the cause of advancement to duck the awkward issues. Instead we need to address them conscientiously and vigorously.

The necessary mind—brain link probably comes within known physics laws which at present remain hidden from view simply because of current practical limitations and gaps in our theoretical understanding (as was the case for so many centuries regarding the body's energy fields). All we can say with our present state of knowledge is that a thought potential somehow excites an electromagnetic response which can then act at a distance.

We have already seen that the human energy field can damage or disrupt computers, watches and other sensitive electronic equipment. I wrote about this in *The Allergy Handbook* and suggested that allergy sufferers seemed to have far more powerful electromagnetic 'auras' than most people. As a spectacular demonstration of this human energy charge, an experiment was conducted at the Menninger Foundation.[6] Exceptional subjects were suspended in front of a large wired copper wall and were shown to give off very substantial electromagnetic fields. These fields were easily capable of disrupting micro-electronics and therefore capable of attracting reads on an EAV instrument.

A cadre of scientists have taken the view that if quantum theory is the best explanation of reality we have at present, then it should take account of mind and consciousness and the part these play in phenomena. Professor D. F. Lawden at Aston University, Birmingham, England, is among those who think that systems which are dependent on the observer state, that is which include consciousness in the nature of the construct, are especially worthy of study.

Several of the Virtual Medicine diagnostic and therapeutic techniques I have detailed in this book are just such examples of psycho-physical states displaying quantum characteristics. Lawden has gone so far as to draw up modifications of the basic equations of quantum mechanics, to allow for possible disturbing psychic effects being introduced by the participants.[7] This has also helped to clarify what constraints to 'reality' there may be, when recognizing there is no absolute or autonomous state. In this, Lawden likens quantum science to the philosophy of Irish bishop George Berkeley (1685–1753), one of the so-called

British Empiricists. Berkeley's basic premise was that all matter and material form has no meaning whatever outside the mind. It might be there, but how could we ever contact it without mind?

To accept Lawden's argument would put ideas and sensations as the primary events, and matter (particles, energy) as secondary participants; this is exactly where our Eastern forebears left our cosmos 4,000 years ago. We have gone through the convolutions of supposedly superior scientific method, right up to the minute and beyond, only to end up where intuitive gifts and metaphysical *knowing* took us a long time ago!

Casebook: Male, 40 Years

Finally, in case this review of objectivity should have suggested that the Vega test or any EAV is of doubtful worth, let me cite a case from the files of world-class EAV specialist Anthony Scott-Morley of Poole in Dorset.

The patient had complained of persistent discomfort in the region of the liver. Routine laboratory examinations by the family doctor had revealed no abnormality. Orthodox treatment including anxiolytic drugs had, not surprisingly, failed. The private opinion of the referring doctor was that the patient was neurotic and would benefit from psychotherapy.

Vega testing showed a stressed liver which was balanced by the ampoule *aflatoxin*. Aflatoxin is a highly toxic fungus commonly growing on mouldy nuts, especially peanuts. Scott-Morley asked the patient if peanuts had any significance for him. The patient expressed great surprise and started to cry.

It emerged that he had been employed as a truck driver and had some months earlier transported a truckload of peanuts to England. On arrival at Customs the consignment had been condemned as mouldy and unfit for human consumption. Yet the driver had, not unnaturally, consumed many handfuls on his journey across Europe.

Treatment using the Aflaxotin nosode resulted in prompt and permanent relief of all symptoms.

CHAPTER 6

BIORESONANCE THERAPY

We have considered so far how the patient's energy field is paramount, and how disturbances in that field may give rise to disease. A novel idea which evolved in the 1970s, piggy-backing new technological possibilities, was to use modifications of the patient's *own* energy emissions as a means of eliminating disharmony and morbidity. If we can somehow use electronic machines to strengthen the healthy energies and at the same time eliminate the unhealthy ones, whole new therapeutic possibilities open up. This was the line taken by Dr Franz Morell and led along a parallel development sequence to the Vegatest.

The term 'bioresonance therapy' (BRT) has come to mean therapy with the patient's own oscillations. This differs somewhat from the EAV approach on two main counts: first, that one need not identify the cause of pathological oscillations, and second that the counter-agent or means of eliminating the wrong energies need not be some exterior agent, such as a medicine, but can be accomplished by means of modulating or cancelling the unwanted signal, while at the same time strengthening the 'good' energies. We could introduce the term *electronic homeopathy* for this class of healing.

ELECTROMAGNETIC SIGNALS

Pathological electromagnetic oscillations are active alongside normal oscillations in the body of every patient. Indeed, even healthy individuals certainly have some element of such disharmony but, as Lakhovsky suggested, if the energies of the normal cells are stronger than the pathological energies, then health can be maintained (page 21). On the other hand, if Lakhovsky's 'war of energies' goes ill for the tissues and cells, the resulting disturbance of the dynamic equilibrium will lead to disease, even cancer and death. The important point is that the electromagnetic signals from a diseased patient contain all the information needed for therapy, if only we could successfully decode it.

Morell's idea was that we do not necessarily need to decode it, if only we can identify which signals are the problem. Ideally there would be some kind of filtering process to divert the pathological energies, which could then be altered and used to modulate the disease process. The problem is to know which are the bad energies, among the huge volume of information traffic and 'noise' going on round a living organism such as a human body. Fortunately, harmonious energies do tend to be similar from person to person. These are the dynamic energies. Any impinging signal which is fixed is very likely to be non-biological in nature; in other words, harmful.

THE MORA MACHINE

Morell went to work, with his son-in-law Erich Rasche, and together they developed a device now known as the MORA machine (MO from Morell and RA from Rasche). Rasche, an electronics engineer, reports that it was some time during 1976 that Morell handed him over 500 small metal washers. These were colour-coded and, according to Morell, had the 'information signal' imprinted in them of homeopathic potencies. The idea was to use these for remedy testing, along the lines of EAV. Plexiglas sheets holding 100 washers each were made; 10 such sheets would store 1,000 remedy tests.

In fact, nothing directly came of this idea and it was not until the advent of computer technology a decade later that this dream of storing a large number of 'information signals' came to fruition.[1]

However, this got the two men started on research and development, together with bio-physicist Ludger Mersmann, and what they came up with in 1977 was a machine which certainly changed the face of future medicine. We are still only two decades into its development, and so it has far from fulfilled its potential yet. But, scientifically speaking, the principle is simple and sound; technologically it is straightforward; and therapeutically it has proved its usefulness time and time again. As the energy medicine paradigm advances, the MORA machine will grow in stature. Already there are a number of copycat and derivative devices, including the BICOM, which is discussed later.

What the MORA machine basically does is enhance harmonious oscillations to help the tissues overthrow the noxious process, and inverts pathological signals, which effectively cancels them out.

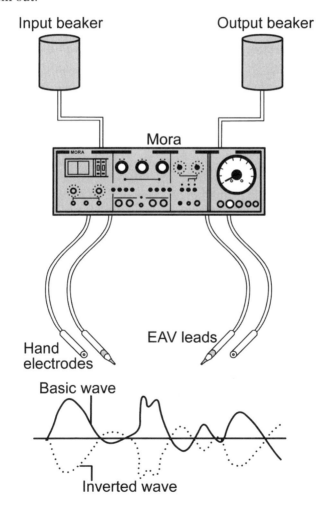

A little more physics is needed here. A wave form has peaks and troughs, as the signal 'oscillates' or varies in intensity. To invert a signal means to put peaks where there were troughs, and vice versa; this effectively results in zero energy, since one cancels out the other (see illustration below). It is very simple to arrange this electronic process. In fact Rasche also arranged that all signals could be passed through to the patient, unaltered; the harmonious signals could be amplified (but would not, logically, be inverted), or the harmonious energy, combined with inverted pathological energy, could both be amplified if necessary.

The input signals from the patient are picked up directly from electrodes held in the hand, or from foot-plates. These are delivered to the machine and modified in various ways. The resulting output or therapeutic signals can be 'played back' through the same electrodes, or via a probe. As in 'Basic Therapy' described below, the input signal may even be taken from a little of the patient's body fluid, such as saliva or blood.

In addition to the electronic apparatus necessary to make these arrangements, the MORA machine is also fitted with an EAV device, since practitioners of BRT are almost invariably involved with EAV, so close are the two disciplines.

However it should be pointed out that the MORA machine probably has more in common with Abrams' Oscilloclast and Boyd's Emanometer than with EAV.[2] Other possibilities offered by this family of machines include the use of low light frequencies, filtered and modulated, which are then played back electronically through skin electrodes, or the use of direct light enhancement (compare this with the machine described in Chapter 9).

A USEFUL EXPERIMENT

Experiments on animals can be revealing. One uses animals not only because doing so throws up fewer moral implications, but also because in doing so one can exclude likely psychological factors.

In a 1985 study using Syrian hamsters, benefits from bioresonance were clearly seen which could have no placebo basis. One group of hamsters was treated with bioresonance, while the controls were left untreated. All other factors, such as food, heat and lighting were kept constant. Various parameters were studied, including red cell count, a differential leukocyte count (thus giving lymphocyte totals), weight and quantitative food hoarding.

The treated group became more lively, their defence and flight reactions were faster and their coats were smoother than those of the controls. Food hoarding, a species sign of health, was considerably higher in the treated group than in the controls.

Among the haematological parameters tested which were significant, the treated group showed a marked rise in lymphocytes, which is equivalent to an increase in immune function and longevity.[3] The protocol, though simple, was impeccable and the results convincing.

Veterinary bioresonance has since become a reality. Animals are said to be particularly rewarding and responsive subjects. It is just as effective with very large animals, as with smaller species. The only difficult group are the very hairy patients!

BASIC THERAPY

The methodology of BRT is relatively simple. Before starting with a therapeutic regimen using a device such as the MORA machine, it is customary to carry out a pre-treatment or so-called 'Basic Therapy'. This means to enhance harmonious energies and invert pathological ones, so strengthening the patient's resources. This can be very important with chronically sick and weakened patients, who want to be in good shape to receive the main therapeutic energies without being knocked over by them!

The patient provides a little saliva which is put into the metal beaker on the input side. This beaker is in effect a receiving device, rather like a radio aerial; the signal is led away through a lead, to be amplified and modulated within the apparatus. Other 'input' samples could include skin scrapings, nasal secretions or vaginal and rectal swabs – in fact any bodily tissue or fluid.

Settings on the machine allow simple choices such as amplification, inversion and filtering. For children it may even be desirable to attenuate the signal somewhat. A few minutes of this pre-treatment is all that is required.

VOLL MERIDIANS

The MORA specialist then goes on to test individual meridians, keeping a note of the readings at each Central Measurement Point (CMP). This is much in line with Voll's method; balance is taken to be anything between 45 and 55. Again, too high is inflammatory and too low means degeneration. Indicator Drops (IDs) are seen, exactly as you would expect.

But here is where bioresonance enters. With bioresonance it is possible to alter the emanations being collected by the probe at each main pathology point (most abnormal reading or biggest ID), using the amplification, inversion and broadcast principle. The modern MORA has various settings which allow the practitioner to focus on different bands or 'windows' of frequencies. He can then take the incoming signal and make three basic changes: amplify it; invert it and amplify it; or filter out the pathological signals. The way this is decided in practice is by playing each modulation in turn and seeing which brings the point back *nearest* to the ideal 50.

A treatment would then consist of playing the therapeutic signal through the patient for several minutes. The body cannot respond well to the intensity of a constant signal; it becomes refractory. Instead the therapeutic message is broken up into parcels. A fixed number of timed units can be spaced out with pauses between. Empirical tests indicate that 3 seconds of signal followed by 1 second of pause is probably optimum. In this way the full treatment energy is received without resistance by the tissues.

Scorch Marks

At the time of writing I do not use a MORA device, but leading British EAV specialist Stan Richardson has remarked to me that after a BRT session it is often possible to see scorched hand prints on the pickup and output electrode bars. This is especially noticeable if the bars are left untouched overnight and allowed to 'develop' photographically. Moreover, the output side has a different pattern to the input side. Stan feels that there may be some kind of coded message here, if only we could decipher it, akin to the Kirlian photograph (page 47).

This also brings to mind Lakhovsky's theories of cellular radiation and the 'spontaneous radiographs' of C Nodon (page 22).

ALLERGIES

One unusual aspect of the MORA machine, not shared by other EAV apparatus, is the ability to modify allergy signals. I have always argued that allergy is basically an information-field signal, rather than a biochemical process, as explained on page 66. Because of this little-known fact (i.e. that allergy is basically an information-field signal) there is the potential to modify the patient's receptivity to the harmful energy of an allergen.

This is also, incidentally, a good demonstration for those who remain sceptical about the whole process now being described. If the patient's allergen is placed in the beaker and the signal therefrom is played back electromagnetically through the output electrodes, the patient may experience symptoms. It is remarkable that the signal for wheat can provoke, say, an attack of wheezing in an asthmatic. If not, turning up the amplitude of the signal is very likely to do so. This verifies the existence of the allergy and proves that it is *not* a biochemical or immune process, whatever conventional medicine says. It allows us to show once and for all that every substance has a unique energetic signal and that this can harmfully interact with our endogenous energies. No chemical or fluid changes position or enters the patient's body, yet symptoms are triggered!

Treatment of allergies may be effectively carried out by inverting the input signal. It is not easy to see the logic of this but it does seem to work; indeed, in my opinion it is one of the best available uses of the MORA family of devices. Perhaps the body is being electromagnetically reprogrammed using the 'anti-allergy' signal, which can then be incorporated into the energetic dynamics. Treatment takes place weekly, with gradually increasing numbers of timed units, rather like the old immunological allergy protection known as hypo-sensitization, where the dose increases until the body can learn to tolerate it. From then on it protects the body in much the same way that any antidote would.

As an amusing aside, this process can be carried out on other substances. If cheap rough whisky or wine is placed into the tray, and then signals from it are inverted and played back *into the bottle*, the resulting drink is unquestionably enhanced. This claim never fails to attract laughter and disbelief from audiences; yet even the most incredulous of sceptics is usually impressed by the happy result. Blind tastings show that there is indeed a difference.

MERCURY AMALGAM

So much has been said about mercury toxicity from dental amalgams that it would be superfluous to debate the issue here. More is said about it in Chapter 12, along with other more important and up-to-the-minute theories.

MORA therapy does offer a new approach to this problem. Whereas one should remove fillings and so eliminate the source of contamination, this does not remove established tissue deposits, which are often considerable. One can try to use chelation agents such as DMPS (dimercapto-propane sulphonic acid) and DMSA (dimercaptosuccinic acid), which bind with the mercury and so eliminate it through the kidneys. But even this has potential dangers, since DMPS actually binds with neurological tissue and so cannot eliminate brain deposits. A better plan is to use the MORA playback facility to invert and counter the mercury signal, in much the same way as is done with an allergen. Rasche claims that this actually enhances the excretion of amalgam compounds.

The EAV part of the device can be used to establish exactly what heavy metal burden is present in the patient's body. This can then be used in the input beaker and the signal inverted, amplified and thus neutralized. Generally, Rasche recommends that the heavier the mercury burden, the higher the amplification needed. This seems to be logically sound.

Treatments are carried out twice a week for 3 to 4 weeks. Drinking copious soft water helps the ion elimination process and this is mainly effective at the time of therapy. In Rasche's words 'The excretion process continues until the earth's natural magnetic field realigns the elementary particles of the remaining amalgam.'[4]

OTHER APPLICATIONS

There are clearly very many possible applications for this energetic approach to health. Some which have had particularly gratifying results include infertility, where sperm count and motility have been seen to increase markedly after BRT; extensive burns, where non-invasiveness is a strong point; healing of bones; eye problems; tinnitus and gynaecological problems. Children appreciate this treatment modality, since no pain is felt and their natural apprehensiveness is soon appeased. The child or infant can sit happily on his or her parent's lap while therapy is administered. ECG electrodes (the kind with rubber elastic straps) can be adapted as electrodes for very small babies.

Bioresonance therapy is especially useful in the management of addictions, such as tobacco and drugs. It is very helpful to an individual going through the unpleasant withdrawal phase to have harmful energies filtered out and natural, health-boosting frequencies amplified. Obviously this does not eliminate the need for the patient to make a clear and determined decision to *stop* indulging their addiction. But by forcing the excretion of toxins and balancing yin-yang energies, the misery is much reduced.

Thus, after a general Basic Therapy, the addictive substance is placed in the input beaker and passed to the patient inverted and amplified, exactly as described for allergens and toxins above. It is essential to prescribe a simultaneous forced excretion therapy, including copious amounts of water, teas, enemas and liver cleansing. Vigorous exercise, lymph massage and depuration saunas are also helpful where possible. Homeopathic drainage support and organ stimulants may also be indicated (see Chapter 7).

Finally, an aggressive vitamin and mineral programme is required, to help the body nutritionally overcome the toxins present and to ensure renewed healing and tissue repair. Withdrawal symptoms are very stressful to the organism and adrenal cortical function is often at maximum revs. High doses of vitamin C in the 10–20 grammes range are also useful as a short-term detoxicant.

Even where the regime proves quickly successful, it is recommended that the patient attends regularly for many months, to reinforce the determination to quit.

PAIN

'Pain is the cry of connective tissue caused by blocked energy'; so the saying goes. This maxim of Dr Weichel was often quoted by Voll. It emphasizes that pain is not really a local manifestation, even though the triggers may appear to be. Morell found benefit from treating the ends of those meridians (Ting points) which pass through the pain area, starting with the mirror-image points on the side opposite the painful area.

This can be followed by picking up signals from the pain area and, after inversion, playing these back to the tissues somewhat distal to the disease area. *Increasing the amplitude of the inverted signal effectively pushes it deeper and deeper into the tissues.*

If pain is intensified during the treatment, this may not be a reason to stop the therapy. The practitioner must decide each case individually, but there can be a degree of beneficial intensification before the pain finally eases off. Sometimes physiological changes can be seen in the skin, such as a white patch becoming visible. This area should be made the target of output therapeutic energies. Treatment is continued until the skin resumes normal colouration.

Casebook: Male, 6 Years

This boy developed an astrocytoma, which has a very bleak prognosis. The consultant neurosurgeon had recommended chemotherapy. The parents, who were Buddhists, had rejected the idea and decided their child would die gently and with dignity, if that was to be. They prayed. Even better, they also took him to see a MORA therapist.

By this time the boy was in a desperate state and was so weak and wasted he had to be helped to walk into the clinic. The practitioner took blood and subjected it to the inversion and amplification process described; just a few minutes for the first visit. The child was sent home with homeopathic support therapy along the lines described for mesenchyme therapy in Chapter 7. Then, by gradually building up the timed units of treatment, once a week and then, eventually, once a fortnight, the lad was soon feeling well. A few months later he was able to resume athletics and playing rugby football.

The practitioner, who could also use a Vega machine, tested and found no remaining tumour signal, but there was a focus which was cystic. At about this time, the parents (without telling the MORA practitioner) took their son back to the original consultant. He was surprised to even see the boy alive. As is often the attitude, he was dismissive and said 'We must have been mistaken in our diagnosis.' This angered the parents, who were naturally incensed at the idea of their son being subject to chemotherapy based on a shaky diagnosis. But the old scans were brought out and re-examined: there could be no doubt. It was a tumour all right. With persuasion, the parents allowed a re-scan which showed that only a cyst now remained where once the tumour had been. The MORA practitioner has a copy of the letter from the hospital confirming this in his files.

This was a very satisfactory result for Virtual Medicine. Incidentally, the specialist never asked what the miraculous treatment was or showed the slightest interest in learning about it. He goes on giving chemotherapy to his patients.

BAND PASS DEVICES
Certain improvements in the basic MORA procedure suggest themselves. A competitive device, developed by former US MORA representative Hans Brügemann, addresses some of the issues. It has taken advantage of available computer technology

and is accordingly dubbed the BICOM (BI-ological COM-puter).

It has around a thousand pre-programmed case handlings, with pre-set frequencies and timed units based on the pooled knowledge of many practitioners of the MORA school. Among the problems which can be dealt with in this easy way are:

Problem	Pre-set Programme
eye inflammation	(520)
bladder irritation	(490)
diabetes	(45)
muscular pain	(630)
hacking cough	(540)
wound healing, stimulating	(931)
selenium metabolism, stimulating	(804)
and so on...	

101 is the so-called 'basic programme'. A BICOM practitioner is also offered the possibility of entering and storing their own favourite programmes. This is certainly an advance over the 'manual programming' of the MORA machine and an obvious benefit of computer technology that lends itself to the situation.

But the chief technological advance the BICOM boasts is the use of a *band pass*, a cyclical passage of a narrow 'information window' up and down the scale from 10 Hz to 150,000 Hz. This innovation is based on the observation over many years that therapy works best if oscillations are returned in a relatively narrow range. Otherwise the cellular dynamics may be given too much to deal with.

Couple this with the discovery by Cyril Smith at Salford University, England, that effective bioresonance therapy results in an immediate response, whereas less appropriate or detrimental energies take some time to develop the adverse effect. It makes sense to move rapidly over the ground and give short bursts of therapeutic signals, rather than linger as with the older method.

Thus we have a number of new options in the BICOM, over and above returning all frequencies simultaneously:

1 Only a small part of the frequency is returned, in a selected range, usually chosen by the operator.

2 A range of frequencies is swept just either side of a central set figure. Technically this is known as 'wobble'. The amount of wobble can be varied but still operates within a relatively narrow range.

3 The whole end-to-end range is swept automatically, concentrating on one part at a time, but covering every possible allowed frequency.

It will be seen that only option 3 actually covers all possible frequencies, though not all at once. It may be important to operate over the whole range; since no frequency is transmitted for long the chance of developing adverse effects is almost zero, whereas the benefits, as Smith showed, happen almost instantly. Furthermore, the patient may respond favourably to several different frequencies; in fact commonly does. This ensures these secondary beneficial zones will be visited too; and yet overall it saves the operator time.

A Brief Critique

Much controversy has surrounded the BICOM, some of which, if valid, should rightly be aimed at the MORA machine too. Part of the attack on the BICOM's performance has come from rival manufacturers, such as Vega. The latter claim to have special electronic sensing equipment which has examined the output from the BICOM and shown it to be worthless and not what is claimed. Perhaps this should be seen mainly in terms of a marketing offensive, rather than the purest of scientific motives.

One thing is certainly true: BICOM comes under the anti-radionics legislation in the US and encountered hostility from the authorities. The American public, it seems, needs protecting from funny waves, even though the US Food and Drug Administration claims these waves are not there!

The EAV device incorporated in the BICOM is perfectly straightforward and cannot be challenged legitimately by Vega.

Also the inversion and amplification channels are simple and unarguable electronics manipulations.

The logic and empirical science behind the band pass is perfectly cogent to me. It is notable in this respect that the MORA people have responded by introducing the band-pass facility into their own latest machine.

It is only the pre-programme facility of the BICOM that can be separated from the other aspects and targeted for special criticism. I doubt it is so important, since most BRT practitioners have their own views on suitable treatment programmes.

My own unease comes from the performance of the filter or separator, which is absolutely critical to BRT. If your filter lets through the harmful oscillations, the theory is lost. We have no standard against which to judge what is a pathological signal. I indicated above that any fixed vibration is unlikely to be physiological in nature, but other than that it is little more than speculation what a disease oscillation behaves like. Brügemann defends his separator vociferously by pointing to an experiment which showed that temperature drop in healthy patients, caused by subjecting them to the information signal of mercury in the input beaker, was effectively blocked by it. Without the protection of first passing the signal through the separator, subjects experienced an alarming fall in temperature of almost 2 degrees Centigrade within 30 seconds; the experiment had to be discontinued because of heart fibrillations.[5]

My own view is that such an experiment is rather unethical if you believe your own story about negative oscillations. But it also seems to me that Brügemann fails to make his scientific point, since this only shows that the machine can single out mercury signals. It does *not* show it is capable of discerning all good from bad among the huge totality of ultrafine oscillations of the body, as is claimed. *What it does show, which is helpful for my text, is that energy signature oscillations of toxic substances have great impact on biological systems*, exactly as Jacques Benveniste believes (see page 112).

Until the manufacturers stop hiding behind proprietary secrets and tell us what they are using in the separator, we cannot properly evaluate their ideas. Perhaps time and further research will clarify matters for us all.

RESISTANCE TO BRT

A number of factors are recognized to impair or block the benefits of BRT. These have been observed empirically over the years and form a basic list of resistance factors to any kind of therapy.

1 The place of therapy is geopathically stressed.
2 The patient's home or workplace is geopathically stressed.
3 There is a tooth focus or strong amalgam stress (see Chapter 12).
4 There are hidden psychological factors preventing success, which would include the practitioner's own doubts or scepticism.
5 There is a nutritional deficiency (*no* therapy works well in the present of nutrient deficiency).
6 There are hidden toxins, parasites or allergies present.
7 Allopathic drugs have a blocking effect. Even alternative therapies can sometimes interfere with each other.
8 The cables are damaged or the electrodes are not cleaned properly (energy disturbance can be carried over from the previous patient).
9 There is interfering scar tissue.
10 The therapist is insufficiently skilled or knowledgeable at what he or she is attempting.

SUMMARY OF BIORESONANCE THERAPY

Hans Brügemann of the Brügemann Institute, which manufactures the BICOM machine, has nicely summarized the chief precepts for understanding bioresonance therapy. In conclusion I give here a modified description of these:

1 In and around the human body there are electromagnetic oscillations. These oscillations are superordinate to the biochemical processes going on in the tissues and are the real control mechanism of tissue function.

2 As well as physiological oscillations there are also pathological interfering oscillations in every person, caused by
toxin overload, injury, infection, unresolved disease processes and psychologically negative states (so-called emotional toxins).

3 Both natural and pathological oscillations can be picked
up from the skin surface (antenna effect) and led to a suit-
ably tuned therapeutic device.

4 The mixed oscillations from the patient can be modulated in three main ways: (i) healthy signals amplified; (ii)
pathological signals inverted (and thus cancelled out); and
(iii) filtered, to separate the desirable frequencies from the
pathological ones (the latter are, of course, eliminated in
this process).

5 No technologically-generated artificial frequencies are
needed; only oscillations from the patient which have
been modified as given in 4. The basic aim is to strength-
en the good oscillations and eliminate the unwanted
ones.

6 The body takes its cue from the modulated therapeutic
signals and continues to produce enhanced physiological signals and appears to reprogramme itself, so that in
future a renewal of the pathological signals is guarded
against. Thus the treated harmonious levels of electromagnetic energy go beyond the merely temporary stage of
treatment sessions.

7 Beneficial changes in the energy field are followed by a
subsequent modification and improvement in biochemical function and physical structure.

8 BRT is successful when the body's own endogenous regulatory forces reassert control and lead to normalization
and maintained health.

CHAPTER 7

BASIC TREATMENT MODALITIES

It is time now to consider the medicinal therapy which is integral with EAV and its derivative, computer electro-dermal screening technology (see Chapter 8). In general this type of therapy is based on bio-information and energy; these therapeutic substances could therefore be termed 'Virtual Medicines' in line with our overall theme.

To understand the place of this remarkable form of treatment it is useful to look at a categorization of different forms of therapy:

1   **Invasive Methods**
Surgery, lasers, moxa therapy

2   **Biochemical Methods**
a. Inorganic (e.g. minerals)
b. Organic (e.g. herbs, drugs, vitamins)

3   **Energy Methods**
Electro-magnetic waves, Reiki, acupuncture,
 bio-magnetism, sound, music, colour therapy, homaccords

4   **Information Methods**
High-potency homeopathy, Bach flower remedies,
gem therapy, electrical bioresonance, nosodes and sarcodes.

THE ELEMENTS OF HOMEOPATHY

Almost all practitioners of EAV use what is known as complex homeopathy. To understand its precise advantages it is necessary first to clarify the basic nature of homeopathy. Today it is largely forgotten that this was once a major system of treatment taught in over 25 per cent of US medical schools and that, until the arrival earlier this century of patentable allopathic drugs which could be marketed for huge profits, it enjoyed a sound reputation and was widely practised, both in Europe and the New World.

With the coming of the drug boom, however, there emerged a new supposedly scientific paradigm based on laboratory testing on animals and clinical trials, particularly the double-blind sort. Alternative methods, or more traditional (older) approaches, were re-evaluated as 'not scientific'. Even simple remedies such as good food and rest were more or less rubbished in the stampede for newer and better 'magic bullets'. The attitude which today pervades conventional medicine is that what the treatment of disease needs is something to oppose or crush the unruly process. There is no concept of nurture or helping Nature to perform the cure. Indeed, Nature's generous wisdom is often abused or over-ridden, as in the case of chemotherapy or commando surgery for cancer.

Even less do many modern doctors understand that the disease process is necessary; it is a natural complement to the exigencies of life. Without the fight-back response, or what Hippocrates called *ponos* (the bit that hurts!), we would be overwhelmed by our hostile environment. Acute disease is actually the process of throwing off unwanted challenges. Usually this is successful. But by untimely interference with the process of resolution – by administering chemical suppression therapy, for example – we are simply driving the toxins or insult underground, where they will emerge later as a more chronic illness.

Homeopathy does the opposite. Far from being a powerful antagonist of disease, it actually mimics and *uses* the disease process to get the cure!

The name homeopathy comes from 'homo-' (same) and 'pathos' (disease, as in pathology). There is a famous Latin maxim: 'Similia Similibus Curentur', which translated means 'Like cures like.' Although the idea has been in use since Hippocrates' time, and the great Paracelsus also wrote comprehensively of it, it fell to German physician Samuel Hahnemann to organize the key principles of homeopathy into a cogent scientific thesis, which he did in his great work *The Organon of Rational Medicine*, published in 1810 (he was 55 at the time).[1]

An example of this so-called 'law of similars' is that substantial doses of deadly nightshade (Belladonna) produce a clinical picture almost identical with scarlet fever (a once-common form of strep-tococcal tonsillitis which doctors hardly ever see these days). The scarlet fever patient has a, bright red rash (hence the name), burning hot, dry, headachey, maybe even delirious, with wide staring eyes and extreme restlessness. Hahnemann found that if he administered Belladonna to a case of scarlet fever, the results were quite beneficial, sometimes even dramatic.

Potentization

But Hahnemann didn't stop there, and this is where homeopathy indeed seems strange. Hahnemann found that if you *dilute* the active substance, the treatment becomes more effective. The more dilute it is, the more powerful the remedy seems to be. This applies even when the original substance is so dilute there can be no chemical molecules left. Hahnemann called the dilution process *potentization*, since it manifestly made the treatment more powerful.

The apparent illogicality of intensification-by-dilution is what excites so much hostility from conventional doctors. They seem to have a silly fall-back logic which argues: *'It can't work, and therefore it doesn't'*. In fact the results show otherwise. There is an ever-increasing number of scientific trials being published that show homeopathy is an effective and safe alternative to drugs in many conditions. Even so, an editorial in the *Lancet* which accompanied a paper showing that homeopathy worked could not resist sniping with the comment that Hahnemann's theories were 'inherently implausible'.

In fact there is nothing implausible whatever about potentization. It merely requires that one finds the right model. Instead of thinking in terms of the concentration of bio-chemical substances, one has only to think in terms of an information field and realize that this is how homeopathy works. The medicine is carrying a message which knocks out the disease 'similar'. The medicine gets better through dilution, simply because we are diluting out what the technical people call 'noise', meaning the extraneous and unnecessary information which interferes with the message we want carried to the tissues.

But how is this information field conveyed? To understand the mechanism better we have to examine the properties of water, so vital to the life process and bio-energies.

The Peculiar Properties of Water

Every schoolboy and -girl knows that water is a molecule consisting of two hydrogen atoms and one oxygen (H_2O). This molecule has a bi-polar charge – that is, a positive charge at one end and a negative charge at the other. Overall these cancel each other out (making the molecule electrically neutral), but close up this property of electrical polarity has consequences. It means that water molecules can act like tiny magnets, with north and south poles, and 'tag' together in what are known as clusters.

These clumps of molecules are capable of carrying electromagnetic information, rather like signals on magnetic tapes or disks, and it is this peculiar characteristic of water that has immense importance for life energies.

It also has great meaning for therapeutics, because information can be carried to the tissues using the most obvious transporter: the body is made up of almost 70 per cent water. Not only that, but the right sort of energetic information will reach all parts of the whole organism virtually simultaneously.

Unfortunately, but hardly surprisingly, this also means that body systems are susceptible to outside electromagnetic disruption. Nearby electrical fields and even celestial events, such as sun spot activity, can influence the health and dynamics of body tissues. Indeed, popular science author Lyall Watson makes the point in his book *Supernature* that, because of our susceptibility to radiations from space, it is possible to provide a scientific model for the ancient belief system of astrology.[2] We have also seen the rise in the belief that external energy fields, such as high-tension electricity cables, can lead to leukaemia and other unwanted conditions (see chapter 10).

To demonstrate the capability of water for retaining information, spectral analyses of homeopathic remedies have been carried out. The resulting graphs of several homeopathic potencies of Belladonna are shown in the figure below. It should be noted that, according to physical science, dilutions of D23 (one-in-ten dilution repeated 23 times) or higher cannot possibly contain any chemical residue. What is measured is an energetic information signal. Even at high dilutions (D30 and D200), frequencies above the positive line are recorded, meaning that *the solution is actually transmitting information.*

This cannot be explained by merely substance-based think-

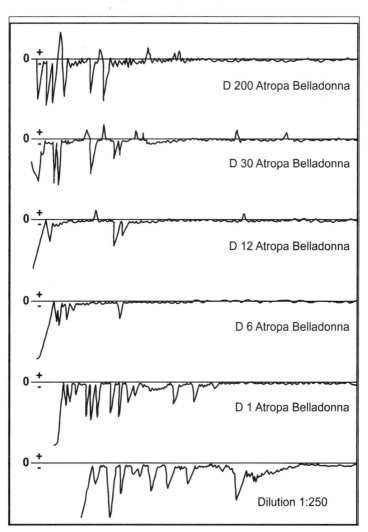

ing. There is no 'stuff' or mass present, though in fact it should be explained that school-level physics leads us to consider mass too simplistically. Scientists now recognize 'weighable' matter, which has a rest mass; but also non-weighable matter – one might resort to calling it 'virtual matter' – which has only energetic properties and no detectable rest mass.

Whatever is in the 'solution' or residual water after the chemical has left, it carries recognizable energetic properties. It can interact with the tissues and with the disease process, to effect a cure. It does this by resonance – that is, striking a frequency chord (as in music) where the two oscillators (or notes) together match up and create a much-intensified response.

Your radio set does much the same thing. The incoming signal is very attenuated but when you tune the dial, you are altering a resonator (the amplifier) until it matches; at that point the signal becomes much stronger and can be used in a modulating electrical circuit, without it being drowned out. In other words, the information (broadcast) is singled out from the surrounding 'noise'.

Thus there may be no Belladonna carried by the water, but its 'radio transmission' is still present and will resonate with scarlet fever, or any similar combination of symptoms. In 1988 Professor Jacques Benveniste published a now-famous paper in *Nature* magazine, reporting experiments which showed that extreme dilutions of water solutions of an antibody could still evoke a biological response long after the active substance was diluted away, *provided the solution was agitated after each dilution.*[3] Non-agitated solutions produced little or no effect. This pointed clearly to transmission of information via some kind of water-organizing process.

Benveniste was bitterly attacked by his peers and even denounced by Sir John Maddox, the then-editor of *Nature*, who had first commissioned the article. For such an affront on the narrow-minded tenets of science Benveniste lost his government funding and his laboratory was closed down. There were even some attempts to prove he had perpetrated a fraud, but in the end this was toned down to hints that his work was not reproducible by others. Such are the vagaries and fashions of science, as Albert Abrams learned (see Chapter 1).

Classical vs Complex Homeopathy

It is sad to report that controversy has broken out even among homeopathic practitioners. There are two factions: the classic homeopaths, practising in the manner of Hahnemann, and those who use what is known as 'complex homeopathy'. I will briefly address the arguments which seem to be creating the rift so that, in looking at the issues, the reader may learn more about both disciplines.

The major difference is that classical homeopathy argues that there must be only one correct remedy for a patient at any one time. It has to be said that there is no scientific or logical basis for this supposition, merely that 'Hahnemann said so,' but to insist upon it as doctrine risks becoming inflexible and out of step with newer developments. Complex homeopathy on the other hand, as you may suppose from its name, means giving multiple remedies at the same time; or only one remedy, but in a range of several different potencies (called a Homaccord).

But there are more subtle differences in philosophy and method between the two fields.

In general, the complex homeopaths use far lower dilutions, closer to what one might call biological values. Classical homeopathy, on the other hand, hots up at around the 30th centesimal, which means a substance diluted 100-fold repeated 30 times (100^{30}); it can go to MM, meaning diluted 500-fold repeated 500 times (500^{500}). To put this into perspective, from 24C (24th centesimal) onwards the dilutions are so enormous there can be no physical substance left.

Complex homeopaths, on the other hand, are quite happy with mixtures that contain 2X, 3X, 6X, etc., meaning a 10-fold dilution repeated 2, 3 and 6 times respectively. Complex homeopaths also tend to use a great deal more of diluted tissues and disease material, which we might call 'isopathy' though this word has little real impact. What this means is not so much 'treating like with like' as using 'same to heal same' (for example, healthy pig pancreas for pancreatic disease, Tonsilla for tonsillitis, Carcino-mium for a lung cancer, and so on). This will be explained more fully below.

Buckshot

The result is that complex homeopathy tends to be less of a one-hit miracle and more of a gradual attrition of the disease process, over a space of several months. Whereas a classical homeopath will stop the remedy the moment it is seen to produce a sig-nificant result, a complex homeopath smiles with satisfaction and adds another two months' prescription to the therapy pro-gramme.

I bring up this controversy in some detail simply because it strikes at the heart of what we mean (or believe we mean) when we talk about homeopathy as being an 'energy medicine' or based on resonance and information fields.

If we believe our own explanation, then complex homeopathy ought to make the more sense of the two. We are talking about energy signals or information patterns resonating or interacting with sympathetic frequencies in the diseased patient. Therefore if there are a number of frequencies or a 'spread' of energies (like buckshot) at around the right magnitude, there will be more chance of successfully hitting the target. The unwanted reso-nances, which find no counterpart in the body, should have no interactive effect whatever. They just go away.

Classical homeopathy, one remedy at a time, it is true can pro-duce very impressive results. But if the practitioner is mistaken in the choice of remedy, *or chooses an unsuitable potency*, there may be little or no result. This means added delays and suffering for the patient, while the practitioner tries something new.

There is another simple, all-too-human appeal in complex remedies. If we doctors are honest with ourselves and others, the reality of daily clinical practice reveals that we are far from per-fect. With the exception of those individuals with outstanding memories it isn't possible to carry a full working knowledge of all potential remedies. A busy homeopath will often settle for a similar (near enough) rather than a true 'similimum' (exact remedy).

This lack of precision in choosing the similimum results in less effective therapy. Complex remedies are designed, at least in part, to accommodate for this lack of precision.

Complex homeopathy is sometimes called the 'German system', though in view of Hahnemann's nationality one could argue that *both* are the property of that great intellectual and cultured race.

In conclusion, it must be pointed out that all complex homeopaths are flexible enough to use classical remedies in the classical manner when these seem appropriate. We accord great respect to Hahnemann's teachings; but are not restricted needlessly by them.

MESENCHYME THERAPY AND THE MATRIX

In the absence of any objective measurable change at the structural or chemical pathological level, doctors are reluctant to consider 'real' disease and think instead of psychiatric or functional disorder (meaning disordered function of the mind; a euphemism for madness or delusion).

But there is another domain or theatre of disease, which, although ignored by the powerful financial lobby which controls modern medicine, has continued to be researched quietly in Europe and the former Soviet bloc for most of this century. We may term it the 'humoral' nature of disease – that is, disease manifested as a result of disruptive imbalances in the quality and content of the fluid medium in which our organs and cells are suspended. Two central figures in the development of this model, which is also sometimes called Homotoxicology, are the clinician Dr Hans-Heinrich Reckeweg and Professor Alfred Pischinger, the father of modern histochemistry.

The fundamental concept is that of homo- (auto)toxins accumulating in the interstitial (support) fluid and tissues which we call the mesenchyme or 'matrix'.[4, 5] Toxin here does not simply mean pollution or waste matter from cells, but includes the 'memory' of disease and the residues of malfunction and stasis. But I would like to challenge the received wisdom. I suggest that the importance of the biochemistry of these toxins is actually secondary to the deterioration in the ionic energy-conductive properties of the collagen matrix. Remember from Chapter 2 that Georges Lakhovsky predicted that the accumulation of interstitial toxins would cause alterations in electromagnetic oscillation potential, which would alter conductance and resistivity and mean that cells could no longer vibrate at their inherent healthy frequencies.

We shall return to this concept of the intercellular matrix and its variable dielectric status in Chapter 11. For the moment let's just say that what is clear is that there is far more interstitial matter than cells which comprise organs. Thus, in terms of volume alone it makes a great deal of sense to pay attention to this fluid matrix. Yet it is barely mentioned in the medical school curriculum and doctors continue to graduate with no more than a passing knowledge of this vital energetic domain of our bodies.

Far from being what is left when you take away the 'important' structures, the connective tissue matrix is the basic regulation system of the entire organism. Without it the organs could not function in a concerted whole. The matrix is to the organs of the body what the engine, gears and wheels are to the body of a car. A harmonious and well-functioning matrix is synonymous with good health.

This matrix has three obvious functions: nutrition, defence and repair. It carries out these functions in response to a whole gamut of input stimuli, whether energy, hormones, osmotic gradients, electrical impulses, immunological signals, neurotransmitters and, of course, any toxin-irritating presence.

What Reckeweg correctly perceived was that if Pischinger's matrix becomes clouded and sludged up with toxins, then there is a cumulative process of degeneration and decay, leading towards advanced pathological conditions, notably malignancy. The same message as Lakhovsky's. The organism works less and less efficiently until resistance is overcome. Finally the processes of pathology take over and run down the machinery towards death. By the time cancer growths appear, the end may well be close. Reckeweg coined the term 'homotoxicosis' for this sequence.

What homotoxicology does is best thought of as de-polluting

the matrix. The skilled use of appropriate complex homeopathic remedies can cleanse or reverse the decay process. It often means using toxin signals, presented homeopathically in the form we call *nosodes*. This drives out the disease process, though unpleasant reactions can appear as the reversal process gets under way. To prevent this we use drainage remedies which speed the elimination of toxins, as described below.

Reckeweg called this cleansing of the matrix and reversal towards a healthy state 'regressive vicariation'. I regard it as a potentially misleading term; I would prefer '*pro*-gressive vicariation', since it gives the idea of improvement. But Reckeweg's chosen expression calls attention to the fact that we are rolling disease backwards, reversing into earlier and better levels of health.

Hering's Law

This reversal of the disease process described by Reckeweg is associated with an older and well-established healing law. It was formulated by the 19th-century American homeopath Constantine Hering, but it applies to many healing disciplines, not just homeopathy. It is a truly great insight into the healing of disease and should be taught in letters of fire to all who aspire to comfort and mend our fellows.

Hering's Law states that, in the course of healing a disease, recovery takes place in three clearly defined ways and that these are signs of meaningful recovery:

1 **Healing is from inside to outside.** Thus a runny nose is an improvement on colitis or asthma. Do *not* diagnose 'rhinitis' and try to prevent the nasal mucus! The response is a healing process and *not* a new disease.

2 **Healing is from top to bottom.** Thus a skin rash will clear from the head first and lower limbs last. Keep going!

3 **Healing takes place from the most important organs towards the least important**. Thus irritable bowel could be a sign of therapeutic response from mental illness. You are drawing the disease from the mind into the body.

There is another very important and related aspect to this, which is that during the process of recovery the disease sometimes 'rolls back' through time: symptoms that came last go first; symptoms that preceded those may reappear for a time before they in turn vanish. A child who developed asthma and then migraine may well go temporarily back to asthma when put on an effective remedial programme (this also fits rule 2). It's like putting the mesenchyme 'car' into reverse; you have to go back through all the old familiar landmarks you passed on your way to 'Disease-ville'.

This observation is often tacked onto Hering's Law, though Hering himself did not phrase it so. Reckeweg may not be the first person to recognize the back-track phenomenon, but he was the first to give it a name, albeit the rather clumsy 'regressive vicariation'!

NOSODES

I have hinted that probably the key therapeutic agent of mesen-chyme therapy is the *nosode*. A nosode is a homeopathically-prepared sample of disease tissue or biological toxins. These samples are negative energy signals of substances which hurt or poison the body, or dangerous tissue. For example Carcinomium, made from cancer tissue, is very hostile to the body, as you would expect. Any disease-producing virus, bacteria or parasite would automatically make a nosode; Dr Edward Bach, famous for his flower remedies discussed shortly, actually made some of the first-ever bacterial nosodes by potentizing vaccines, still known as the Seven Bach Nosodes.[6] Modern advances in the field of EAV and beyond have made it quite clear that pesticides, heavy metal poisons, electro-pathic stress, medicines and numerous other stressors all have the essential character of nosodes.

Nosodes are potentially strong remedies and may provoke an illness in response to their administration. Even though the measles or TB may not be present, except as a virtual signal, the body still reacts as if the disease was in progress. The tissues fight back. The patient feels bad once again; we call this a 'healing crisis'.

Drainage Remedies

Notwithstanding Hering's law, we solve this problem with the use of what are known as 'drainage remedies'. As the name implies, drainage remedies are substances which can provoke speedier toxin removal, whether by stimulating the kidneys, liver or other excretion pathway (diarrhoea is seen by holistic practitioners as nothing more than toxin-flushing and often comes on in response to a treatment). We can categorize drainage according to organ: pancreas, liver, gut, etc. Or we can grade it according to power: mild, gentle, medium, forte and 'ultra' preparations.

It is said that almost any pathological or nosode preparation is capable of working as a drainage remedy, if the dilution is right. This will happen if it is not too forceful (lower potencies) and does not provoke more quickly than it cleanses. One of my patients joked about 'taking her diseases in water'!

It might seem tempting to administer the strongest drainage remedy possible, to give a good flushing to the system. But that is to think like a drug-prescribing physician. All energy medicine is conceptualized on the principle of the so-called 'minimum dose'.

What does this mean?

Adey's Window and Arndt-Schulz's Law

Elementary-school science drums into us the linear or quadratic relationship and we are taught that if a quantity of some substance has a particular effect, then larger amounts will perforce induce a greater effect. But this is often not so.

There are very good biological reasons for the magic of the minimum. If the body is subjected to too strong an input signal, this often has a negative rather than a positive effect. This can be likened to turning up a radio set so loud that it begins to distort. The extra volume is counter-productive and the programme broadcast will be heard better by turning down the volume to a more comfortable level. Overdosing is the way in which many drugs work.

I am convinced that much allopathic medicine is simply poisoning out some part of our physiology; for example, painkillers poison the full working of the nervous system.

Virtual Medicine practitioners have come to understand that the biological information field is paramount, and that the field only needs to be modulated slightly for there to be a major change in output. This is summed up in another holistic principle known as Arndt-Schulz's Law, which applies to homeopathic prescribing but again also to many other interacting living systems:

- A small stimulus will provoke positively
- A larger signal has no further effect
- A very large signal actually has a suppression effect.

W. Ross Adey of Loma Linda University showed this effect experimentally while studying calcium influx in irradiated animal brain cells. He showed that the brain cells not only responded to quite specific frequencies (approx 10 Hz), but did so only at extremely low intensities.[7]

There was, in effect, only a very tiny spread of values in which the optimum effect could be detected. Outside that range either nothing happened, or function was suppressed. This gives us a new term, the *Adey Window*, meaning an effective low-level band or response-slot. Adey received the Hans Selye Award for this holistic insight in March 1999, at Montreux in Switzerland.

Specificity

It is important to note that nosodes are not necessarily given only for the disease to which they relate (for example giving a 'flu nosode in a case of 'flu). In fact that is to underestimate and miss the importance and applicability of this new therapeutic range. Empirically it has been found by Voll, Schimmel and others, that certain diseases associate with particular nosodes. Conversely, some nosodes come up time and again as trouble-makers in many different conditions. Childhood vaccines are particularly notorious in this respect. I think we can go some way towards answering the mystery about where the present post-war epidemic of allergies has come from. At least part of the reason is the childhood vaccination programme, dropping toxins on the immune system, spleen, etc., which then results in malfunction. The child may

avoid the whooping cough or diphtheria, only to suffer with many
more obscure and difficult-to-treat symptoms later in life.

I myself prefer to use homeopathic 'vaccination' in which the
body is accustomed to the noxious agent, using very small safe
doses. It is safer, painless, cheaper and does not have the same
side-effects as true vaccination. (Lest you fear it won't work, it is
interesting to note that in the last great diphtheria epidemic in
Glasgow, just before the advent of antibiotics, over 50 per cent of
the children died with conventional therapy, yet not one fatality
occurred at the city's homeopathic hospital).[8]

Here are some examples of the diversity of effects of nosodes,
though the full reference range of many hundreds of items is a
matter of considerable learning and remains the intellectual property of a well-trained practitioner.

Disease Condition	Nosode Indication
acne	tuberculinum, bacillinum, psorinum
arthritis	streptococcinum, staphylococcinum, apis mellifica, variolinum, vaccinium, influenzinum
breast cancer	tuberculinum, medorrhinum, carcinosin, syphilinum, variolinum
diabetes	parotidinum, diphtherinum, tuberculinum, bacillinum
migraine	diphtherinum, variolinum, vaccinium
prostatitis	tuberculinum, diphtherinum, pertussin
sciatica	influenzinum, staphylococcinum, streptococcinum
warts	medorrhinum

One can reverse the starting place and view each nosode as a
polyvalent remedy – that is, capable of reaching out and de-ener-

gizing many different disease conditions. Thus:

Nosode	Useful in Treating
Herpes (all)	arthritis, canker sores, spleen, shingles, heart, nerve, pancreas
Morbillinum	hypertension, multiple sclerosis, neurological disorders
Syphilinum	swollen knees (especially in women), brain cancer, heart valve disorders, prostatitis, chronic gynaecological problems
Typhoidinum	intestinal complaints, liver, gall bladder, spleen, heart
Varicellinum	arthritis, myocardial disease, multiple sclerosis, cranial nerve palsies, shingles

MIASM

A miasm is one of the most powerful influences in health and disease I know, yet the least acknowledged or understood. The word was introduced by Hahnemann, but I prefer to think of it as a 'genetic toxin', since this term gives a far clearer idea of what we think we are dealing with. Basically a miasm means a shadow or disease 'imprint' which is inherited down the generations.

All observant doctors are aware that disease and disturbance tend to run in families, and can be likened to a kind of family blight. This is not to mean a specific replicated genetic disorder carried by the genes such as, for example, haemophilia or Freidrich's ataxia. The sickliness can manifest itself in many different ways, each individual suffering differently from the others in his or her family tree but all bound by the commonality of being a somewhat weakened or unhealthy bunch.

This idea may seem to be an attempt to revive Lamarck's discredited theory of evolution, which said that an organism's responses to environmental stressors could be passed on to offspring. This is now held not to be true; the Darwinian/Mende-lian dogma reigns, which states that only the factors carried in the genes can be inherited. Rigidity of this degree sounds suspiciously like yet another road-block in scientific thinking; a fashion that will one day have to be exposed to common sense and revised.

To Hahnemann a miasm was something more in the nature of a primitive illness, a throwback. He named three in particular: *Syphilis* (or *Luesinum*), *Sycosis*, and *Psora*. Briefly, *syphilis* has ulcerating tendencies; *sycosis* (meaning from gonorrhoea) is con-gestive, leading to deposits and tumour formation; while *psora* is a protean disturbance which relates to functional imbalances of all kinds.

Psora is said to have formed in the time of the Plague (the Black Death).

Antoine Nebel and Henry C Allen added *Tuberculinum*, which many practitioners now regard as the pre-eminent miasm, presumably since it is but one generation removed from today's population stock.[9] Among the fall-out diseases from this inher-ited toxin one can list asthma, eczema, hay fever, food allergies, chronic sinusitis, migraines, mental illness of various kinds including retardation and subnormality, irritable bowel, colitis, heart trouble, diabetes, Hodgkin's disease and even leukaemia.

Leon Vannier added a fifth, which is the Oncotic (cancer) miasm. It is characterized by changes in body odour, warts, excrescences, sores that refuse to heal and a sallow skin, some-what like that of malignant cachexia.

It is also fashionable to consider the emergence of at least two new miasms: Candida and Chemical Sensitivity; Sugar Glut may very likely become a third modern miasm. I suggest we call the Candida miasm, if we can agree there is one, 'Mouldy'.

I introduced the term 'mouldy patient' in my book *The Allergy Handbook*[10] and it seems to me a far bigger issue than just Can-dida; the patient becomes sensitized to a wide variety of moulds and yeasts. Unquestionably it is brought about by overuse of antibiotics, made worse by our obsession for refined carbohydrate and sugar, which results in a great deal of unnatural fermentable matter in the gut.

May we say then what a miasm is? I think in the light of modern understanding of energetic medicine it is possible to go beyond Hahnemann's hypothesis and say we are surely dealing with some kind of transmittable information field with its accompanying energetic disturbance. It appears 'etheric' or non-material in quality, but that is because hitherto we have not had the electronic means to search in the outer energy shell, except by dowsing. The fact is, miasms show up repeatedly on comprehensive testing of the electro-dermal screening (EDS) sort (see Chapter 8). We know they are there. Treatment consists of giving the homeopathic similar most exactly pertaining to the shadow. EAV and remedy testing can help us to identify and treat miasms with greater accuracy than ever before.

Casebook: Male, 10 Years

From the age of three the patient suffered from repeated vexatious sore throats and ear trouble. He fell steadily behind other children his age in scholastic performance. His tonsils and adenoids had been removed (no improvement) and finally his parents were told by an ear nose and throat (ENT) surgeon that the trouble was caused by allergies and the boy would suffer from this all his life.

Analysis showed that the predominant stressor was TB miasm and an acquired measles toxin. The indicated miasm and nosode were started and continued at appropriate repeat intervals over several months.

The ear and throat condition cleared up rapidly and has never reappeared. The boy's mental and physical slowness, which had been such a worry to his parents and teachers, soon abated and he was able to hold his own with his peers.

THE STUDIOUS MONK

Former head of a monastic order, Simon Goodrich, now an alternative practitioner in Oxford, has worked extensively on historic miasms. Goodrich has identified a number of obscure miasmata and post-infective dyscrasias, along with recommended treatments, which I find most helpful (dyscrasia is a general term for a body disorder, which derives from the old theory of mixed "humours": Greek *krasis*, mixture, hence bad mixture). Here the theory is of an old (but not necessarily ancestral) infective disease process which lingers. A list of the fifteen predispositions, with an historical estimation as to when the particular strain of this condition was prevalent, and in which society, follows here:

GOODRICH'S LIST OF HISTORIC MIASMATA

15) **Cytomegalo-virus (ME):** Spread via cotton trade from USA. Emergence in approximately 1900. Immunity acquired around 1990.

14) **Tuberculinum Kent. (tuberculosis):** Spread through shipping routes in British Empire. Emergence in approximately 1650. Immunity acquired around 1800.

13) **Baryata Acet. (gonorrhoea):** Spread through silk trade with Iranian civilization (Arabia). Emergence in approximately 1600. Immunity acquired around 1750.

12) **Endorid (cholera):** Spread through spice trade from Ceylon, the Ceylonese civilization. Emergence in approximately 1500. Immunity acquired around 1650.

11) **Arsen. Sulph. Rub. (syphilis):** Spread through the jute trade with Bangaladesh, The Mughal Empire. Emergence in approximately 1500. Immunity acquired around 1650.

10) **Lycopus Eur. (The Black Death):** Spread through the fur trade with Turkestan, The Ottoman Empire. Emergence in approximately 1400. Immunity acquired around 1600.

9) **Cobaltum Nit. (The Plague):** Spread through the porcelain trade with Ming China. Emergence in approximately 1200. Immunity acquired around 1400.

8) **Aesclepias Inc. (pneumonia):** Originated in Europe, and prevalanet within the Frankish Empire. Emergence in approximately 600. Immunity acquired around 750.

7) **Droleptan (typhoid):** Originated in Babylonian Empire. Emergence in approximately 900 BC. Immunity acquired around 800 BC.

6) **Apium Grav. (fungal infections):** Originated in Egyptian Empire.

Emergence in approximately 1200 BC. Immunity acquired around 1100 BC.

5) **Urinum (leprosy):** Originated in Hebrew society. Emergence in approximately 1400 BC. Immunity acquired around 1300 BC.

4. **Cornus Flor. (impetigo or scall):** originated in Canaanite society. Emergence in approximately 2200 BC. Immunity acquired around 2000 BC.

3) **Pectinum (uteritis, inflammation of the womb):** Originated in Pheonecian civilization. Emergence in approximately 2600 BC. Immunity acquired around 2400 BC.

2) **Ornithogalum (meningitis, cerebral palsy):** Originated in Sumerian civilization. Emergence in approximately 3200 BC. Immunity acquired around 3000 BC.

1) **Cuprum Met (genital herpes):** era unknown

[*Goodrich's remedy is shown with each condition*]

Controversially, Simon told me his researches led him to believe that we each carry a number of miasms and this impacts our survival. The body's energies can become locked up in fighting the miasms, with adverse consequences for long-term health. With four miasms present, the individual is unlikely to survive (succumbs in infancy to childhood illnesses or teen disasters, such as leukaemia); a person with three miasms will make it to adult life but die early (heart attack at 40- 50 for men, breast cancer same age range for women); with two miasms, that's good for survival to 60- 70 years; the lucky person with only one miasm should make it through to 70- 80 and beyond. All this, unless you are lucky enough to meet a skilled homeopath or good EAV specialist!

BACH FLOWER REMEDIES

One cannot consider energy medicine, particularly the information-in-water-alcohol kind, without giving some consideration to Bach's flower remedies. These are superb information medicines of the virtual sort and a great gift to the healer from a humanistic but strange man.

Despite the Germanic sounding name, Bach (pronounced like batch) was actually of Welsh origin, born near Birmingham in 1886. He practised homeopathy in fashionable Harley Street in the 1920s. After 1930 he gave up his successful practice to study plants and trees and their psychological effects, culminating in the publication of the book *The Twelve Healers and Other Remedies*.[11] Today there are 38 remedies in all, ranging from gentian, through wild oat, to oak.

One outstanding remedy called 'Rescue Remedy' (a mixture of Cherry Plum, Clematis, Impatiens, Rock Rose and Star of Bethlehem) seems to have a special place. I have seen it effective against shock, trauma, children's hysteria, travel sickness, rashes and even bees refusing to pollinate. It is one of medicine's truly *great* remedies and should be in the emergency cupboard in every home. A word of caution, however: it is a shock remedy and if you take it when not in shock it can predispose unpleasant shock-like reactions. Never use Rescue Remedy prophylactically (as a preventative).

Bach was what is sometimes called a 'sensitive' – that is, a person who has the gift for unusual psychic perceptions. I have noticed that surprisingly many of these people, for all their gifts, are not very healthy. Bach was no exception and died tragically young. Maybe their gifts are the *result* of being out of focus with the rest of us. I have seen this effect so often in my allergy patients; I soon became aware that feeling unreal and depersonalized has a certain transcendent aspect.

What Bach came to investigate was the way in which psychological attitudes prevented the normal healing and recovery process. It is usually forgotten today, when his remedies are in fashion for every kind of psychological hang-up, that what he originally proposed to treat were merely the barriers to healing.

He carried out his investigations by touching plants or the dew which settled on flowers and noting the emotional feeling it gave to him. He collected the coded botanical information by shining sunlight through the petals onto a brandy and water stock (sunlight method); or by boiling down the plant to create a concentrated extract or tincture (boiling method). Only one remedy, Rock Water, is not botanical in origin but is exactly what its name suggests and comes from mountain streams.

Bach remedies are unquestionably bio-informational in character, which is why they are reviewed here. They work mainly at the etheric or trans-dimensional level, and are in every sense a 'virtual remedy'. A person sometimes has only to touch or hold the bottle to get an emotional release. Your author actually burst into tears on picking up a book describing these remedies; I tell this only because I think it says more about the remedies than about me! Make of this strange occurrence what you will.

One theoretical objection might be the concern that what applied to Bach and his other-wordly persona would not necessarily apply to the rest of us, or at least not in the same manner. However, this hypothetical problem has largely been taken care of with the passage of time; the remedies today enjoy enormous popularity, and world-wide sales attest to their astonishing efficacy.

CLINICAL APPLICATIONS

I can only echo Bach's original view and say that, in my own electronic diagnosis and therapy system called the Acupro (see Chapter 8), I find I sometimes need to add one or more flower essences to the treatment tanks before the Indicator Drop will vanish and we know that the therapy programme will succeed. It is axiomatic that much disease has a psychological element and that unless this is addressed, even by something as gentle as a coded flower message, the patient may have limited recovery.

Casebook: Female, 37 years

Dr Sam Williams tells a remarkable story of a woman patient who had been severely traumatized by a road traffic accident several years before. The emotional impact was, to say the least, unnerving. Ever since, she had been unable to leave her home without being wrapped in heavy blankets against traffic noise and blindfolded, so that she could not see anything connected with cars or roads.

In this pathetic state she was driven to his office and unwrapped, looking very miserable and dishevelled. His Acupro system sang out the flower remedies, including Mimosa, which is 'fear of known things' and the patient went home with her formula, unconvinced.

Despite two decades of EAV experience, no-one was more surprised than Sam when, next morning, the woman drove herself to his office alone, dressed to the nines, and handed him the bottle back in person, saying 'I don't think I need these any more Doc, but thanks!'

She was on her way to her first shopping spree.

In conclusion, Bach has given rise to a whole culture based on flower essences. At least two additional schools have emerged, one in Australia using Pacific Flower Remedies, and the other from the West Coast of the US, the so-called California Essences. Notable is the Flower Essence Society founded in 1979 by Richard Katz. Doubtless there will be more and more expansion as other adepts add their own contributions.

IMPRINTING

This review of the main available remedy modalities for EDS and Virtual Medicine practitioners would be incomplete without describing a sort of trade secret called 'imprinting'.

Dr Franz Morell, the MO- of MORA (Chapter 6), discovered that sometimes during the course of BER medicine, the patient would actually recover if the remedy was 'played back', like a recording, into the patient's tissues, either through the bar electrode or directly via the acupuncture point through which the necessary data was accessed. Very occasionally just being exposed briefly to the remedy while it was being tested was sufficient to produce a therapeutic result. Although the benefit could sometimes last a considerable time, these responses were usually of short duration, often disappearing as soon as the remedy signal was removed from the circuit and the point retested.

But Morell discovered in his experiments that if the chosen remedy oscillation was amplified 8–10 times and then played back, the result could last for weeks, months or even indefinite-ly.[12]

This is basically what the MORA machine does. The rest of us, who don't use one, have to adopt some other means of attaining the same result. This leads almost naturally to the idea of *imprinted* medicines, which can extend the electronically-derived treatment process once the patient has gone home.

An imprinted medicine is one in which the supposed therapeutic electromagnetic message, derived from the Acupro library or similar sources, or a real sample on the input honey-comb, is transferred into a mixture of water and brandy. In other words, instead of giving the patient Echinacea, we play the information signature of Echinacea into the remedy bottle and give the patient that instead.

Lest you think the whole idea absurd, let me tell you that many of the cases reviewed in this book were treated in this way. The very dramatic story of Ed Butler of the Platters (page 140) was treated with only imprinted remedies, since I carry no nosodes of 'flu virus. The machine detected the disease and told me what would eliminate it.

We talk about the individual 'vibrational signature' of substances, herbs, homeopathics, enzymes and other beneficial substances. It ought to be quite logical and indeed scientific, if we really are dealing with nothing other than energy signals, to be able to transfer the energetic signal to a carrier fluid or other medium. I have already explained that the peculiar properties of water and brandy mean that these are especially suited to carrying transferred electromagnetic signals.

We can call this electro-homeopathy.

CAUTION

In view of what has just been stated, it would be remiss of me not to point out a potential danger. If we can imprint the 'signature' of a substance in liquid, it follows that the same would apply even regarding unfriendly or toxic material. Many years ago at an advanced think tank, I heard a proposal that boiling water in an electric kettle or using electric heating rings to cook our food might impart what we ate or drank with hostile electromagnetic energies (bear in the mind that mains frequency of around 50–60 Hz is particularly damaging to biological systems).

I am sorry to say that I somewhat scorned this possibility at the time (1982). At least I should have kept an open mind. Almost two decades on I have learned enough to know that this is more than a theoretical possibility. We certainly *do* imprint liquids with unintended energy codes. A beer on the top of the TV may have a little of your favourite (or most hated) programme in it! The question which remains unanswered is, can imbibing these imprinted substances have detrimental effects on health?.

I have no idea of the answer. But I would say this: keep all medicines and remedies, even vitamins and minerals, *well away* from any source of electromagnetic radiation, such as computers, TVs and microwaves. Otherwise they will almost certainly be spoiled.

THAT MAN BENVENISTE AGAIN

I have already referred in this chapter to the way in which Jacques Benveniste caused a scandal when he published proof of what came to be known as 'the memory of water' in the scientific journal *Nature*. In fact, in the true nature of science, his work has now neen reproduced at different study centres[13, 14, 15]. He is vindicated (but he didn't get an apology).

Now Benveniste is back with even more radical theories about the energetic signatures of molecules. His more recent work suggests that it will be possible to record electronically the specific characteristics of a remedy or any other substance, such as adrenalin, nicotine and caffeine, or the immunological pattern of viruses or other pathogens. These recordings can subsequently be played back and even transmitted through telephone cables and thus on to the Internet and will have a measurable physiological or remedial effect.

His researches, as before, are meticulously controlled, comparing the effects of a "digitized remedy" with the authentic substance, using digitized water (no specific imprint) as a control. So far, Benveniste reports that he can only record and play back a message. He and his team cannot yet recognize patterns or identify unknown substances from their recording.

Once again, Benveniste's startling advances have been subsequently confirmed by work at other centres[16, 17, 18]. If this new breakthrough is true, one science columnist wrote in a British newspaper, it will undoubtedly earn Benveniste a Nobel Prize.[19] Well, you can verify the truth for yourself: go to Benveniste's website, www.digibio.com and watch a video of an actual experiment taking place.

The age of digital medicines is on the way! I find it a sad irony that Albert Abrams already did this, in effect, in 1924. But his brilliance has been somehow forgotten as his star fell.

One exciting aspect of the new hypothesis is that it explains the manner in which many remedies or physiological substances have an almost instantaneous effect throughout the organism. This can be much too fast to be explained by humoral or biochemical means. The usual proposed mechanism is a neurological one. But Benveniste's model makes more sense. It also sheds light on the phenomenon of specific biological receptors. The usual explanation is one of a 'lock and key' mechanism; that is, the receptor site has a physical shape which admits only the correct trigger molecule. I have always viewed this as specious and remarked earlier in the book that allergic reactions, or *recoveries due to therapy*, can be so instantaneous as to beggar the normal pathways. Benveniste's proposal of transmitting molecules and 'tuned' receptor sites (like a radio aerial) fits these clinical observations far better. In his view, it would take only a tiny alteration of the receptor to de-tune it, so that it no longer responds.

I am grateful to Benveniste for progress with understanding one of the last major building blocks of the *Virtual Medicine* paradigm. I would also remind the reader of Roger Coghill's comments on DNA and other cell molecules 'transmitting' the body's genetic message, resulting in species-specific growth (page 21).

Western energy medicine, I believe, is *this*, not a make-over of oriental thinking!

CHAPTER 8

ELECTRO-DERMAL COMPUTER SCREENING

We now come to the moment when the promise of this book's title is close to fulfilment. Picture the scene in a 21st-century doctor's surgery. After the preliminaries, the patient sits down in front of a computer display, picks up the passive electrode and the doctor begins to touch the patient's skin at certain of Voll's electro-acupuncture points which we call the central measurement points (CMPs), one on each vessel or meridian. The sensor is similar to the Dermatron but is now hitched to a high-powered desktop PC and the two talk to each other electronically. There is a picture of a hand skeleton; a bright red dot wanders across each digit, beep-beep-beep. After every measurement the

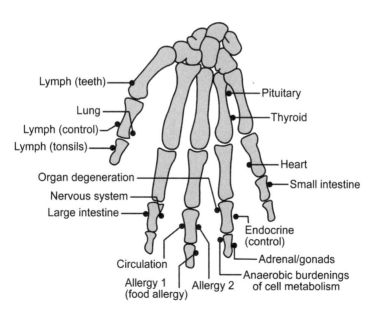

Lymph (teeth)
Lung
Lymph (control)
Lymph (tonsils)
Organ degeneration
Nervous system
Large intestine
Circulation
Allergy 1 (food allergy)
Allergy 2
Pituitary
Thyroid
Heart
Small intestine
Endocrine (control)
Adrenal/gonads
Anaerobic burdenings of cell metabolism

doctor clicks a button and the reading goes into the computer's memory to be stored. We now have an electronic file which can be called up any time in the future and printed out for study or even for the patient to take home a personal copy. Times have changed!

Some things are the same, however. This is still electro-acupuncture according to Voll (EAV): there are two meridians to each finger digit and two to each toe, making a total of 40 readings in all. But when this preliminary stage is complete, by pressing a key the doctor brings up on the screen an attractive coloured graph. It shows all the CMP measurement values; right and left sides are in different colours for ease of identification; Indicator Drops (IDs) are marked as white bands and stand out clearly.

The doctor pauses and looks deep in thought for a few moments. He taps the white marks on the screen and announces: 'Your spleen meridian is down, the endocrine's not so good and something is disturbing the large intestine. The liver is high, which means it is having to detox hard; but there is no drop so no liver damage so far.' He then presses a couple of keys and goes into 'branching', which means that he now studies the spleen meridian in more detail, passing along it point by point, recording all the values and IDs.

You are watching what it says on the screen out of the corner of your eye: lymphocyte function of the upper body – click; serous coating of the spleen (what's that, for goodness sake?) – click; lymphocyte function of the lower body – click; erythrocyte function (that's the red blood cells) – click; reticulo-endothelial system ... the what? You decide this is all very high tech. But the doctor touches a spot just above your left ankle – click, and announces he has finished that step.

Once again, due to the power of the computer, he taps in a key-code and the sequence of measurements is displayed for review as a table showing highs and lows and the size of the Indicator Drops. The 12-point ID which was found on the CMP reappears on SP2, the reference point for 'lower body leukocyte function'. The doctor is satisfied that this is probably what was disturbing the spleen meridian. Something in the lower body is producing an energetic disturbance that upsets or overstresses the lymphocyte function down there. This could cause a chain reaction, since we need our lymphocytes for defence.

Really upset lymphocytes could even mean leukaemia. There is a problem. But what?

DATABASE

Next, as I think of it, comes *Dr Kildare Meets Chinese Traditional Medicine in Cyberspace*. The doctor calls up a comprehensive database of disease entities and possible cures. On my own system there are over 25,000 entries. This is fairly typical for software packages of this type.

By highlighting an entry and pressing the return key, the doctor can access the energy signal named there on the screen. He can then compare it with what is coming from the disease zone; he does this by touching Spleen 2 with the probe, where he found the biggest drop. He no longer looks for IDs but is probing to see if there is a resonance. This is shown by a reading at or very close to Voll's balanced reading of 50. This means a 'yes' from the body.

But the doctor still has to make choices: could it be a virus? A parasite? Malaria maybe; that's likely for spleen for anyone who has been to the tropics ... and so on. But he can check his theories very quickly and begin to establish the likely cause of the trouble.

The software programmer, if he is good, will already have programmed in some suggestions which relate to that meridian. For the spleen one would give high priority to testing infectious mononeucleosis, 'flu, Tuberculinum, Diphtherinum, pertussis, tetanus, malaria, Variolinum (smallpox) and hepatitis A, B and C. These would accordingly come at the top of the list.

Gall-bladder would give a different range of suggestions. On my system the first 10 offers (in order) are: cholelithiasis (gallstone), amoeba, streptococcus, staphylococcus, 'flu, Diphtherinum, Variolinum, TB and hepatitis A and B.

The nerve-degeneration channel would put measles and rubella in the first 10; also probably Syphilinum and Medorrhinum (gonorrhoea code), which may be less obvious.

This is a good moment to reiterate that EAV gives one a completely different perspective on the origins and nature of disease. Remember that we are testing an energetic signal. This is not looking for antibodies to the micro-organism or a sample culture to 'prove' that this is what the patient has *right now*. Indeed, it generally turns out to be something *from long ago*. Time and again, when we question the patient, he or she can remember the problem that the machine has unearthed and says is still causing trouble. Sometimes the patient will telephone next day, excited, to say that a parent or some other relative confirms the diagnosis which the patient was unable to remember personally at the screening session. Childhood diseases and vaccinations come up over and over again as underpinning disease in later life. The energy disturbance is still around, provoking trouble years later. The proof of such a contentious remark, of course, is that when you lift the signal, the patient begins to improve!

More of this later.

THE PRODUCT LIBRARY

We can think in terms of a 'library' of signals available to the practitioner to check against. Among the likely categories found in a computer database for this sort of testing are signals of:
At first such a huge database can seem very overwhelming, there

- alcohol products
- amino acids
- ayurvedic herbs
- bacteria nosodes
- chemicals
- biological age
- geopathic stress
- colour therapies
- chakras
- dental materials
- enzymes
- flower remedies
- herbal remedies
- gems and crystals
- hormones
- environmentals
- essential oils
- food allergies
- grass pollens
- habit drugs

- heavy metals
- homeopathics: combinations, drainage, singles
- polychrests *(a subdivision of homeopathics, polychrests are major remedies with great impact and many ramifications)*
- miasms
- minerals
- parasites
- pesticides
- phenolics
- pollens
- sarcodes *(healthy tissue signals used as support)*
- Scheussler tissue salts
- tree pollens
- vaccines
- venoms
- viruses
- vitamins

are so many choices; how is it possible for one brain to take it all in? Actually, it isn't too daunting.

First, it has to be said that no one individual does or possibly could use and come to grips with *all* of it; I mean understand all the possibilities to a professional level. There have to be selections and generally we work to our strengths. My system has chakras listed: I've never even opened this section for a patient, since in all honesty I wouldn't know what to do with a chakra that was out of balance. But I understand nosodes, such as bacteria, viruses, parasites, chemical toxins, vaccines and allopathic drugs, and I 'find' these a great deal, since I am looking for them. As with all EAV systems, allergies and nutritional guidance is a strong point.

The second vital point which brings it within human capability is that computers by their very nature can help a lot when searching, namely breaking things down relentlessly with either-or logic. It is possible to test a hundred possibilities, then halve it and test that, then halve again, and so on. There is a mathematical principle that you can get down to one item with just six, or at the most seven, decisions using this split logic. Thus if there is a single item you want buried somewhere in a hundred possibilities, it can take less than 20 seconds to find it; such is the power of computers.

The really *great* thing about these computer programmes is that they will tell you first: *'Yes there is something in this list of test substances'*. You don't have to waste time searching fruitlessly in sub-folders that are not relevant to the case.

A refinement which is added to the LISTEN system – one of the first such software packages; the name stands for Life Information Systems Ten, and was developed by James Hoyte Clark of Orem, Utah – is that the search is made 'blind': the items on the list are kept hidden from the practitioner until after he has decided which agent is the real culprit or the desired remedy. This eliminates any prejudgement by the practitioner, which can bedevil objective results and is a good answer to criticism that EAV is really just sophisticated 'dowsing'.

However, it needs to be said that in these advanced systems, nothing can take the place of clinical experience on the part of the practitioner. The machine does not (yet) think for us. It does not 'know', for example, that a large bowel ID, with intestinal lymphatic stress and toxic liver burdenings, would suggest a parasite high in the probable list, or that a head focus is likely to be tonsils, teeth and then sinuses, in that order.

ELECTRO-DERMAL SCREENING

We call this investigative process with computer-based Voll technology electro-dermal screening (EDS). With necessary caution, I can state that it holds great promise for the future. Considering that we are merely in the first decade or two of its development, it already surpasses expectation. As more is learned and scientific studies using this approach give us even more insight and understanding into what is happening in disease, then I think we may soon see a time when it is the basis of any sensible medical practice. EDS is a quick, non-invasive and painless method of health screening.

There are a number of systems you might run into, all much of a muchness. I do not wish to become involved in arguing the relative merits of each; cost, software facilities and back-up service would all be part of such an evaluation. But of the ones I have heard of, I can suggest good results from the following: the BEST (bio-energetic stress test) system, LISTEN, Acupro, Avatar and the revolutionary Limbic Ark (page 228). Now the MORA firm have put together a machine which has a computer library and could, fairly, be said to have joined this group of devices. Since it also combines the facility of bioresonance (see Chapter 6) with EAV and a database, it is perhaps the best machine on the market at this time.

For medico-legal reasons, in the US these devices are considered a 'new device' to be used for investigational purposes only. This is a good description. But actually I have found them also educational. One does learn about illness in a totally new way by exploring each case for the consequences which finally led to the onset of disease.

The really critical factor in getting results is not the software but the operator's ability. The most sophisticated device in the world is less than useful if not backed up by the knowledge and skill requisite for using it. It is still fundamentally EAV and is subject to all the difficulties in objectivity found with this approach. We have to be honest and recognize the drawbacks, as well as the strengths.

Tanks

There are many advantages to using a computer, not the least of which is what we call 'the holding tanks'. These can store diagnostic information and useful remedies and return the signal of their contents to the site being skin-tested. My system has eight holding tanks in all. Remedies can be directed into any one of the eight and stored there, to be played back and tested against the tissue, in company with later choices.

These tanks can be switched in and out, which gives us a number of potential refinements. Thus we sometimes see that a remedy is effective on a particular meridian but when later treatments, especially nosodes or stressors are introduced for treating other organs, that the first point becomes unsettled. We can switch tanks or substances in or out until we find which is the culprit. We can test the whole planned treatment regimen against several points consecutively.

A tank behaves just like a honeycomb on the Dermatron or Vega machine. Filters can be put into the tanks and held there for subsequent testing. They also allow us to organize our thinking a little: I prefer to put my flower remedies in one tank, allergy results in another, homeopathics in a third, biological age in a fourth, and so on.

Most systems will allow one to imprint individual tanks to make individualized remedies.

Filters

A wise EDS specialist will take a leaf out of Schimmel's book and call up the Vega filters for tolerance (Ferrum metallicum D800), compatibility (Manganum metallicum D26) and effectiveness (Ferrum metallicum D26). These can be put into tank 1 and remain there as a background filtering process. This ensures that any remedies chosen are likely to be not only effective but well tolerated by the patient and compatible with other aspects of therapy.

Once a reading-stressed area is found, then a remedy programme needs to be found which will relieve the problem. Obviously an effective remedy must be able to eliminate the ID. We are, in effect, interviewing the body's cells and asking the tissues what they want. Operator knowledge is important, but with such a vast database on tap what he knows becomes less of an issue.

At first the budding EDS practitioner will tend to go along with nosodes and other suggestions put forward by the software. But gradually the practitioner learns his or her own path through this database.

As a comment, I have started to use Bach's flower remedies simply because, on many occasions, I could not get rid of the ID until I included these; often more than one at a time, which will incense the purists. The inference is, of course, that all disease has some psychological component. Unless that is addressed there is resistance to treatment, as Bach postulated. Time and again the patient will recognize themselves in the description of the flower remedy or, if not, a close relative will speak for them and confirm how uncannily accurate EDS can be.

A typical EDS machine is capable of potentizing energy signals. Thus if Candida albicans is a reading pathogen, as part of its software capability the machine is able to offer for testing a Candida 4X, 6X, 8X, 12X, 24X and so on. The centesimal scale is also represented (see Chapter 7). Generally these are 'softer' in nature. They are more applicable to chronic or constitutional conditions. My system, the Acupro, even allows testing of a range of 5X potencies, which can be used in correlation with the allergy testing and neutralization system known as Miller's method.[1]

Thus the practitioner can make up his or her own remedy formulas by combining different strengths of different substances (which can be imprinted, as described on page 128). Also supplied are what we call *accompanying remedies*, which are selected for each organ concerned. These give lift and support for the organ and help to eliminate toxins. They are in fact specially chosen drainage remedies (see page 119).

Many proprietary remedy brands are included with these machines, such as Heel products, Reckeweg, Pascoe and Futureplex, to name a few. Here in the USA one could cite the Deseret Biologicals range. Again, practitioners tend to develop prescribing favourites, but it often happens that only one remedy reads 'OK' and this is what the body is saying it really wants, regardless of preferences.

Accuracy

Most EDS systems take advantage of the computer modality to allow the practitioner to set a definition of 'yes' or 'no' when choosing a remedy. Voll's classic 50 is a theoretical mean. Some practitioners will take anything between 45 and 55 as a positive acceptance by the tissues. I prefer to tune mine at 48 – 52, but since the Acupro takes anything borderline as a 'yes' this degree of accuracy can be very inconvenient at times.

The difficult part is getting the probe pressure just right. Too much or too little pressure will markedly alter the reading. I would say that the touch required is every bit as fine as getting a correct note on a violin string.

The Avatar claims to have the advantage that a feather touch is what the system is set up to operate on. This is supposed to be more reproducible, though I do not know on what premise.

Casebook: Male, 57 Years

I was called to see Ed Butler of the Platters singing group. He had just had a massive right-sided stroke, a few days after completing his last recording session. He was now severely incapacitated and sitting disconsolately in a wheelchair. EDS screening showed a major drop on the nervous channel, which was hardly surprising. But what surprised me was that the read was on the *right*. Yet, as everyone knows, the motor nerves cross over before leaving the cranium and the left brain controls the right-sided musculature.

Notwithstanding, I chose to believe what the machine was telling me. I used the right-side as a reference zone. A search for pathogens revealed a loud and unmistakable signal for 1975 'flu. I checked with Ed who, even though it was 23 years previously, remembered clearly having a bad attack and being confined to bed for two weeks. 'That was the start of your stroke,' I told him. In my earlier *Allergy Handbook* I have already pointed out the great potential of 'flu virus to cause considerable neurological damage.

I made up some X-potencies of this pathogen and offered it to the Voll point; it showed a big improvement but the reading was still dropping to a degree. I added some gentle drainage and homeopathic Co-enzyme compositum (a Heel product), to reinvigorate the metabolic process. The read had almost disappeared. Finally, I decided to try flower remedies; including one or two of these did the trick. I gave Ed the remedy the machine had selected for him. In the meantime he was having energetic healing of the 'hands of light' type.

The very next day I had a call that he could move his thumb. Only six weeks into a massive cerebro-vascular accident this was indeed startling. Good recoveries are possible, but we think in terms of 12 – 18 months, not just a few weeks. In any case this was less than 24 hours after starting the 'virtual' remedy.

Over the next few weeks he improved steadily but then pegged. At this point I recognized the remedy was exhausted due to the heat of our Spanish summer, because it had begun to happen with several other patients. I refreshed his remedy, taking the chance to add a couple of items suggested by the repeat test. Once again, the *next day*, I had a call that he was now able to stand on his legs, provided he kept his weight off the weak side. He soon learned to walk and within six months he was back singing in public; an altogether remarkable recovery from a potentially disastrous episode.

I give due credit to the energetic healers, but the immediate response to the remedy indicated by the Acupro is unarguable. Ed's grit and determination were also, of course, major factors.

OTHER REMEDIES

Yet another advantage of the flexible complex homeopathy approach emerges in the EDS domain. It is possible to give 'remedies' of a non-disease modality. For example, we can intervene in metabolic pathways by giving potentized enzyme similimums. Often I find that a person is loaded with toxins and quite sick, with low personal and metabolic energies. It takes quite a lot of internal cellular energy to push out toxins, maybe against a chemical gradient. Thus a vicious circle is established. It may require the use of enzymes of the Kreb's cycle to bring metabolism back up to speed, before the patient can recover. Mixtures such as Heel's 'Co-enzyme compositum' can really help any detox programme by stimulating chemical energy pathways. The patient usually reports subjective increases in energy levels.

We can also administer homeopathically-potentized support signals of substances like essential fatty acids (GLA and EPA), vitamins or minerals. This is not the same as supplementation, which I would always give 'in the physical' as we say. But often the process of uptake and utilization of such nutrient substances is enhanced by the signal 'in the etheric'! It comes back to the subject of resonance; if the body meets something with which it resonates, a new level of energy can be created. The lithium experiment described on page 14 demonstrates this vital principle.

We can beneficially intervene in hormone secretion and response to hormones, either by giving potentized hormones or endocrine gland similimums. If the relevant organ can be stimulated, supplementation may indeed be unnecessary. Thyroidea comp. (HEEL or BHI) is a remedy I have frequent recourse to for treating low energy states, weight problems, putative low thyroid and, surprisingly, it has strong anti-tumour potentiality, since there is a correlation between thyroid disease and cancer. The thyroid has important and generally little-regarded effects in maintaining strong immunity. This is quite logical if you consider that the thyroid is responsible for setting the basal metabolic rate. Often the patient does not need to take thyroxine.

Other possibilities include balancing neuro-transmitters, such as dopamine and serotonin, with consequent benefit to the patient's mental well-being, anti-parasitic programmes and resonance with personal chemical pollution, such as organophosphates or heavy metals.

With the benefits of a data file record it is nice to be able to revisit earlier diagnostic discoveries and compare them graphically or numerically with later progress.

SO-CALLED IMPONDERABLES

Given the essentially informational nature of the VIRTUAL MEDICINE paradigm, it would be hardly suprising that almost any substance can be encoded and checked against the patient's energy body, to see if it is a help or a hindrance to health.

It is possible to check the chakras and balance those which need it; to test colours and use those which suggest themselves as treatments; relationships; even moonlight!

We call these intangible elements *imponderables* (meaning have no substance and cannot be weighed).

Taking the information idea one step further, Dr Vaughn Cook has told me informally that he has carried out tests in which data sets (such as a language vocabulary) were imprinted into liquid as an oscillating signal and then transferred to the subject, using lazer therapy; with the result that the individual scored significantly higher after study than controls which had not been so treated. Cook was keen to point out that the individual must still study the topic. Information imprinting did not avert the need to learn by did seem to improve scores.

We are both eager to repeat this in a formal clinical trial.

I must say this revelation put me in mind of Edgar Cayce's claim that he need only to sleep with a book beneath his pillow to absorb details of what was said in the print. A remarkable claim; but then, Cayce was a very remarkable man.

Apart from being a gifted psychic, Cayce also devized the "bio-battery". It contains no battery but is a kind of mind enhancement machine that creates subtle improvements of mood and definite improvements of memory. The bio-battery is perhaps a kind of "virtual information machine", working on the body's energetic aura. According to Cayce, "It can almost build a new brain"! He said the device could help amnesia, senility, dementia, brain damage or retardation[2]. This is impossible according to the currently-fashionable mechanistic model of consciousness. Memory lost is irretrievable.

But "Memory is never lost," said Cayce. In his view memory was stored outside of the body. In the 1930s this claim was absurd or at best mystical. Now we can see that he understood over half a century ago that the living being was an information and energy field.

CAUSAL CHAINS

I made my reputation as an 'allergy detective'. I've found pathological reactions to all kinds of strange substances, from herbicide on a bowling ball to a husband's semen, via food, chemicals, electromagnetic fields and meteorological phenomena. The recoveries have been very gratifying. I hope I will never lose my knack for this.

But there has always been the nagging question in the background: *why has this person got allergies or intolerances in the first place?* Part of the ongoing controversy over 25 years of my clinical ecology practice has been that it is comparatively rare that these reactions are what I was taught characterized an allergy (IgE-mediated acute hypersensitivity response) when I was at medical school. It has sometimes been a considerable mystery why the patient should react as he does. A type of antibody serum sickness has been proposed, but this is still within the biochemical hypersensitivity domain.

Now at last, since learning EDS, I have begun to find *real* solutions to this riddle. The answers that come up are enlightening, fascinating, almost unbelievable and, sometimes, rather scary (see Chapter 12). I have long thought that allergy was really the *final* result in the patient's problem, rather than the true cause. Now I can see that this suspicion is not only well-founded, but I can get an idea of just how much the patient has suffered, often without realizing it, to arrive at the doorway marked *'Allergy– Enter'*.

We speak today of 'causal chains'; that is, the true sequence of events which led up to the patient's current predicament. The all-important question, naturally, is *Where did this sequence start?* This often opens the door to a new therapeutic plan which, after all the years of distress and illness, has a good chance of succeeding. It can seem like lateral thinking gone mad sometimes, but there is always an understandable logic behind the events, once they are put into some kind of sequence and perspective.

Nearly always, the problem starts in an unsuspected way with an earlier illness which does not properly resolve. Ed Butler's 'flu of 23 years earlier is just one of many examples. The energetic shadow or disturbance remains in or around the body, sometimes for life, unless it is found and eradicated. One is wise to accept what is found and, time and again, the results speak for the veracity of the hypothesis.

I can only say that I have seen childhood illnesses and especially vaccines initiate disease sequences so many times that I am left with a sense of great unease. What can we do to stop our kids getting ill? I don't think we should abandon the vaccination programmes, we don't want a renewal of the epidemics of old. But how can we get round this difficulty of causing chronic health hazards?

I am not sure. But I do know that my concern is shared by many other doctors who have stumbled across this unpleasant truth while performing routine EAV and EDS. I think that part of the problem is that we *treat* the disease when it manifests and thereby block its proper resolution.

A wise old Chinese doctor, Yang Tschau, once said 'Beware of treating the symptoms of a disease.' Yet in Western biochemically-based medicine that is almost all that is done; no attention is paid to the *true* causes of disease, only the causes of *manifestations* of disease. Yet so often the actual disease is the person's habits and lifestyle; the illness itself is only an outward symptom of what went wrong.

It may emerge in time that it is better to leave most illnesses untreated, especially avoiding the use of allopathic medicines, rather than block natural recovery. I firmly believe from my studies to date that to block an acute illness is to risk driving it underground, from where it may emerge years later to cause a more chronic illness.

Another very worrying concern and challenging management problem is the focus. I already mentioned this phenomenon in Chapter 4; dental foci are discussed further in Chapter 12. It is quite clear to the unprejudiced observer that foci can generate problems far from where they are found. There is compelling evidence that toxic and infective matter can travel along nerve channels, as well as along the more obvious blood route (see page 62). In one case the bacterium *Pseudomonas* was recovered from a cervical spinal osteitis in a man who had the same organism in his urine. The likely mode of travel was along the venous plexus of the spinal column. If this can happen at all, it can happen any time!

I become worried if I think of the bigger implications.

A focus may also pose dangers by initiating pathological changes locally, that is without spreading to a remote site. It is highly likely that an infective focus can give origin to a tumour, possibly due to synthesis of carcinogens by bacterial and fungal micro-organisms. We know that *Aspergillus flavus* (Aflatoxin) and common bacteria, such as *E. coli*, can do this. Late Professor of Neurology in Stockholm Dr Patrick Stortebecker makes it clear that a peri-apical abcess is a very typical finding in close proximity to a jaw cancer[3].

NEW CLINICAL PERSPECTIVES

It is right to talk about new clinical perspectives with EDS. The whole view of disease changes. Indeed, it is a paradigm shift, no less. Even the language of healing changes. It is proverbial that Eskimos have around 50 words for snow, since their technical knowledge of its form, texture and properties is so much more detailed than ours. It is the same with the new medicine. *Focus, energetic masking, homotoxins* and *mesenchyme* become the new rhetoric, instead of the names of obscure pathogens and weird little eponymous syndromes which most doctors would have to look up in a textbook to remind themselves what form it took.

One becomes confident, I believe, in viewing disease as non-random but operating to probabilistic laws, governed by energetic phenomena which impact on our physical systems and control them. We are controlled by biological information fields through an energy system; surely this is the way to start looking at disease? Why just mop the floor when you can go back to the leaking tap and turn it off?

Perhaps I can illustrate some of these newer orientations by featuring cases from the files of EDS specialist Ann Smithells, director of the Bio-Tech Health and Nutrition Centre in Petersfield, UK. Ann was a LISTEN user for many years but now has the latest BEST (bio-energetic stress test) system.

Casebook: Male, 53 Years

The patient first attended because of a chemical taste he was experiencing and excreting. His medical history revealed he was taking the medication Sotol for cardiac arrhythmias, he had high stress levels, nausea, headaches, fatigue and lack of concentration.

Ann's initial screening identified Candida, adrenal exhaustion, low zinc and digestive enzymes, plus high levels of toxins in the gall-bladder, prostate, liver, lung and connective tissues. These toxins were mainly heavy metals, probably due to current dental amalgam removal, and very high levels of benzene. The latter was the putative cause of the bad taste.

The patient was given homeopathics and a high dose antioxidant formula to deal with the heavy metal overload and a homeopathic nosode of benzene at 10M and 20X. Four months later he was much improved but there were still high levels of benzene. This forced an investigation into the cause and it turned out to be a leaking fuel pipe in his car, which shunted petrol into the vehicle's ventilation system whenever he pressed the accelerator.

Casebook: Male, 23 Years

The patient attended a year and half after a lengthy tour of the North Vietnam jungle in search of biological specimens. He complained of hunger, significant weight loss, occasional abdominal pain after eating and insufficient energy to participate in sports, despite being a former county tennis player.

Ann identified inflammation of the stomach, liver, lymph meridians (suggesting parasites) and pituitary gland. He also had a high chemical intolerance. A number of exotic parasites were found, together with bacterial encephalitis and high levels of DDT.

The LISTEN system identified the need for 20 different remedies, including nosodes and the miasm Medorrhinum at 10M, and high-dose antioxidants. To complement these therapies the patient was put on a whole-food diet, with lots of organic fruit and vegetables. He was also given a liver support formula, HEP 194 from Biocare, UK.

Within 8 weeks the patient had gained more than a stone (14 lb) in weight and reported his energy was returning to its former levels. Most of the meridians had rebalanced. The liver, which characteristically produces a high reading when detoxing, gradually came down to normal.

This is a patient who had been let down by conventional medicine. It needed a complete rethink from within a different paradigm.

CANCER

It is possible to see cancer coming with good EAV, while it is still just an energy disturbance and sometimes *years* before the actual disease is manifest. Occasionally the EAV cancer-predictive low readings (30 on down) do not show up as expected. It was suggested by EAV expert Anthony Scott-Morley that the tumour may be surrounded by an inflammatory process, which causes paradoxically high readings. However there are a number of warning signs in EDS that would require a high degree of suspicion of cancer, either established or developing imminently. These include readings below 30 on any meridian, multiple large ID drops, high biological age, low immune performance, chronic toxic overload, dangerous foci in the teeth and anaerobic burdenings (meaning that the general cell chemistry is running too slowly and not burning up molecular fuel properly, creating toxins).

Probably there is no better way of summarizing the difference between the methods of the EDS prescriber and the conventional doctor than to review cancer therapy. Western scientific doctors look upon cancer as an invasion; cancer cells are 'the enemy'. Their response is to fight back with as much fire power as possible, in an attempt to slaughter every last cancer cell. The patient's body becomes the battlefield and is otherwise ignored. Yet anyone who has seen pictures of the blasted wastelands around the trenches of the First World War will know that the battlefield comes off worse than either army.

The EDS specialist looks at cancer as the final results of many disease pathways. We are used to thinking of it as a tissue ageing process, where toxins and pathogens have accumulated to such an extent that the body defences can no longer cope. We try to undo the ill-effects of years of negative health, thread by thread.

Douglas Lieber, director of Computronix Electromedical Systems and the inventor of the Acupro system, pinpoints seven main factors contributing to deterioration in health and leading, if untreated, ultimately to system breakdown and the threat of cancer. These are:

1 geopathic stress, centred especially around the patient's bed or daytime chair
2 parasites of many types present in the body
3 degenerative toxic focus, most commonly in the teeth or jaws but also often in the tonsils or pelvic abdominal areas
4 unresolved emotional trauma
5 miasmic influences, from parent to child, passed through the generations
6 radiation and/or electromagnetic exposure
7 personal chemical pollution with toxins such as nickel, cadmium, mercury, aflatoxins (from moulds and fungi), pesticides, benzene, toluene, xylene, formaldehyde, iso-propyl alcohol and 'autotoxins', chiefly from the patient's own intestines.[4]

EDS specialists make no attempts to treat the cancer, only to treat the patient. If he or she is going to survive the intruder, the patient will need a fortified immune system that is capable of closing down the attack. This can only be achieved by detoxing, removing coincidental and distracting pathology, pumping up nutrition and taking remedies known to stimulate immunity. Of course this cannot all be done with homeopathy. I myself give intravenous drips containing high-key nutritional supplements, especially high-dose vitamin C which is a proven safe cytotoxic agent. Dental work and other physical intervention may be indicated.

Most important of all, *the patient must change his or her life, radically*. Cancer is a wake-up call; it means the patient is badly off-balance in respect of all or part of his or her life. Unless steps are taken to remedy toxic relationships, unhappy work conditions and low self-image, then no therapy is going to be effective against cancer.

It is hardly necessary to point out that these are good universal health measures and apply to any chronic disease process. I call it my ortho-immune programme; *ortho* meaning good or best, as in ortho-pedics.

Suitable complex homeopathic remedies that can be considered are:

1. *Viscum* (Mistletoe) in various combinations. Iscador is
Rudolph Stiener's formula. HEEL (BHI) do Viscum compositum.

2. Echinacea compounds, alternating as immune boosters.

3. Glyoxal (very powerful and for intermittent use only)

4. Causticum

5. *Carcinominum* (nosode)

6. Drainage remedies, eg. lymphomyosot (HEEL), galium

7. Detoxing compounds (Berberis, Nux vom, etc)

8. Defense remedies eg. *Tonsilla comp.*, *Discus comp.* (HEEL)

9. Miasms, individually or composite, as in *Psorino-HEEL.*

10. Specific tumour nosodes, bronchus, uterus, cervical cancer etc.

Dental and other foci will need to be eliminated. In truth, it comes back to my old saw that all good health measures are anti-cancer measures.

BACK TO EDS

So to finish, here I will report on an amazing machine in my possession. It's called the Acuvision and was developed by Romen Avagyan from Moscow. Avagyan got his PhD in radio and quantum physics in 1977 from Moscow State University.

I mentioned Gaikin's observation that Kirlian photography flares often appear at acupuncture points (page 49). With the Acuvisions we charge up the subject with high frequencies and high-voltage electronics, which then causes the acupuncture points to become illuminated and visible on the skin. This clearly hearkens back to the emission of Popp's biophotons (page 51).

The points are about the size of a pin-head and can only be seen in a darkened room. It is thrilling and eerie to see the living body behaving like a lamp and throwing out blue light through real skin "pores". Apparently there are many more points than appear in classic texts or even Voll's extended system. It is of note that the Nogier ear acupuncture points stand out particularly well (page 49).

To date the Acuvision is no more than an intersting curiosity but Avagyan hopes to develop it further. We'll see.

LIGHT AS THERAPY

It is important not to forget that light is just another electromagnetic wave form. The fact that we can see it gives us a deep psychological relationship to light; but it is really no different in quality to radio-waves or x-rays. Because of this we can gain a glimpse of what detailed information may be contained in energy form.

Among the earliest writers to advocate the medical use of light were Herodotus, Galen and the great Arabian physician Avicenna. The ancient Egyptians used a type of colour therapy. But the Greeks went further in both the theory and practice of light medicine, using the sun's rays to treat disease in the famous healing temples of Heliopolis (Sun City).

In our own century, Nobel Laureate Albert Szent-Gyorgi, who discovered vitamin C, acknowledges the profound influence of light on our health and states 'all the energy we take into our bodies is derived from the sun.'[1] By this he means that light is turned from electromagnetic sun energy into energized chemicals by the process of photosynthesis in plants. These plant energy substances (food) are subsequently taken in by leaf-eating animals, who are then in turn devoured by carnivorous species. Ultimately, all life energy derives from the sun. It is correct to speak of light as a *nutrient*.

But Szent-Gyorgi took it much further than this. His research concluded that many of the body's enzymes and hormones are functionally sensitive to light. Colour changes can significantly affect the power and effectiveness of these enzymes and hormones. His findings were subsequently verified by researchers Martinek and Berezin in 1979. They found that some colours can increase the activity of enzymes by up to 500 per cent and markedly affect the transport of chemicals across cell membranes.[2] It has even been found that the absence of certain wavelengths in light results in the body being unable to absorb fully all dietary nutrients.

Little wonder, then, that *lack* of light can have severely destructive health consequences. Few people today have not heard of the unfortunate condition of SAD, or Seasonal Affect Disorder. This is a disorder in which the shortage of adequate sunlight during the winter months of a northern climate causes gradual loss of vitality and even suicidal depression. The cure, quite naturally, is to enhance ambient light levels, either by judiciously taken winter holidays in sunnier climes, or the artificial simulation of daylight. This can be supplied by means of lamps with an adjusted output that has the correct natural daylight spectrum of colours (normal electric lighting has far too much of the yellow frequencies and is lacking in red and blue-violet).

MAL-ILLUMINATION

The study of light adaptation in humans and the attendant ills caused by deficiencies or incorrect balance in colour frequencies has gone on apace in the last few decades. We now have the term *mal-illumination*, a concept proposed by John Nash Ott, who works with therapeutic full-spectrum lighting.[3] He compares this term with our existing term 'malnutrition'. Windows, windscreens, eyeglasses and urban pollution are among the factors which alter the nature of the light our bodies receive, by filtering out some of the wavelengths. Mal-illumination is said to contribute to fatigue, tooth decay, depression, hostility, suppressed immune function, strokes, loss of hair, skin damage and even cancer.

Sunlight is therefore vital to our well-being and, in the current climate of ultraviolet scares, this should not be lost sight of (no pun intended). Despite the medical fad for claiming that skin cancer is caused by sunlight, the evidence points in exactly the opposite direction. A paper published in the 7th August 1982 edition of the British medical journal the *Lancet*, based on a study carried out jointly between the London School of Hygiene and Tropical Medicine and the University of Sydney's Melanoma Clinic, found that the incidence of malignant melanoma was far higher in office workers than in those who were regularly exposed to sunlight due to lifestyle or occupation.[4]

When scientific opinion departs from common sense, it is nearly always science that is found wrong in the end. In this case it is *dangerously* wrong! Light simply cannot be both a nutrient and a poison at normal ambient levels.

CEREBRAL PATHWAYS

The fact is that most of today's light therapy work, colour therapies included, is concerned with light delivered to the eyes. It travels the optic pathways and stimulates, among other regions, the hypothalamus, which is part of the endocrine system and thus influences a most all bodily functions. It seems likely, in the light of modern research, that the pineal gland is far from the vestigial organ it was once thought to be but is actually a master gland which regulates the body's circadian rhythms. As befits the 'Third Eye', it is truly light-sensitive and once again the quality of light received is the crucial factor in maintaining the delicate impulses that regulate the fundamental balance of functions and maintain health.

LIGHT TO THE TISSUES

Light is of unquestionable value via the optical nerve route, as the growing body of scientific evidence and clinical experience shows. But revolutionary healing work with light energy radiation delivered directly to the stressed tissues using machines which deliver quantum 'excited' gem substances, such as diamond and sapphire, is one of the most fascinating and promising frontiers of medicine.

Probably the most advanced machine of this type is the Lux Caduceus III (you may also meet as the Stellar Delux), developed by Jon Whale. An electronic design engineer by profession, in the 1980s he designed electronic transducers using emeralds and blue sapphires and used them to cure a number of cases of psoriasis and chronic cystitis. He now runs a busy practice in Devon, England, and manufactures his equipment for world-wide export. He now runs a busy practice in the north of England and manufactures his equipment for world-wide export.

The essence of this approach is that light can be 'stressed' with the characteristics of the gems. The changes to the light are probably at the quantum level and we are unable to perceive them. But the body tissues can detect the changes and react differently to each type of light, in a most remarkable and consistent fashion.

The important point to grasp is that light travels very far into the tissues. The experience of shining a torch through your hand on a dark night will tell you this; even a small wattage of a 3 volt battery torch will make the back of the hand glow red as the blood vessels and deep tissue are illuminated. The Caduceus Lux lamps use high-intensity bulbs. The powerful beam is filtered and focused through lenses and consequently has far more penetration. Whale has designed lamps which house the gems in the path of the light and concentrate it in a useful beam. The whole apparatus is simple to use and, indeed, a number of users are paramedical in status only, yet obtain results that are little short of sensational. Recoveries range from breast lumps to arthritis, eczema to colitis.

AYURVEDIC GEM ELIXIR THERAPY

This whole new science is really an extension of existing ayurvedic gem elixir therapy, which has a long and distinguished tradition in the Indian subcontinent and can be traced back to Egyptian times. Gems are placed into the tincture liquid and the whole exposed to sunlight until the elixir takes on the characteristics of that gem substance. Theory views disease and disharmony as basically colour starvation; the 'excited' liquid of the elixir rectifies the energy deficit.[5]

As Whale explains, the huge bejewelled rings that were worn by Indian princes, nabobs and potentates were not always merely for the display of wealth and self-aggrandisement. Some rings were intended for therapeutic purposes. Such a ring had no back, so that sunlight could shine straight through the precious stone and so irradiate the skin and tissues beneath with beneficial rays (in common with all energy medicine systems, it is not necessary to bathe the whole body in the treatment or remedy in order to benefit from it).

The other major traditional route of administration was using ground-up gem powders. I consider this a very dangerous practice and it is not to be recommended. It is wrong and over-simplifies the case to feel that gems are safe just because they are manifestly not *chemically* toxic or come from an esoteric background. These substances can be very powerful emanators and modulators of quantum electromagnetic force, as we shall see below, and should be regarded seriously as such. Introducing solid substances which perhaps may never be removed or excreted fully from the body, but can go on causing harm if they are the wrong choice, may prove disastrous. Even when we understand these things much better than we do now, it still lacks sensible rationale as these gem powders may pre-empt any possibility of changing modalities as the body's state or disease process alters.

Readers who wish to experiment with gem elixirs should make them up as described above and *not* take the solid form – even if cost is no object!

Gem Science

Unfortunately, this fascinating yet cogent discipline has too long languished and is still little known outside its country of origin. Modern light therapists and researchers such as Jacob Liberman and John Ott seem to ignore it. But with the advancement of science and the ability to translate older methods from a stultifying background into a modern framework and quantifiable results, we may say 'gem therapy' has indeed come of age and will grow steadily in applications in the West.

Despite superficial similarities, this is not crystal therapy. Quartz, amethyst, tourmaline, moonstone and many other commonly used therapeutic crystals the reader may have heard about seem to have little or no value in this 'light-stressing' context.

Nor is it exactly colour therapy. Tests show that the colour of the light is irrelevant. In other words, it is the *gem* which dictates the resulting effect and not its colour as perceived by the patient. This is odd, since the Indian tradition regards the need for gems and their effectiveness as being evidence of colour starvation.

Notwithstanding, Whale adds the colours traditionally associated with each gem (see list below). But he emphasizes that these colour filters could be dispensed with. The gem carries the energy signal. Whale also electronically modulates the gem stones in his lamps with an additional frequency associated with the body's own natural healing frequencies.

What you feel when you put your hand in the beam is a distinct and palpable pressure from the radiation. It is an astonishing thing to experience. Light from the Caduceus III has the power to shine right through the skull or chest and will thus reach all tissues, even bone, though in varying intensity according to its density.

The applications are remarkably diverse. Thus emerald and sapphire, when excited, emit cooling soothing energies which can stop eczema or inflammation dead in their tracks. Focused on the bowel, this represents a totally new method of calming the gut in, say, colitis or diverticulitis. Ruby will energize cells and glands, and Whale asserts it is excellent for rejuvenating tired male potency. Diamond, on the other hand, is stimulating and, mixed with yellow citrine, peps up lethargy and fatigue states such as those which characterize ME, Candida and complex allergy conditions. But too much diamond can cause a patient to lose sleep for several days.

The principal effect of the main gems and their associated colours are shown here:

Gem	Colour	Energy Output and Properties
Carnelian	Orange	*Cooling, moist and harmonizing, anti-allergic*
Chrysoberyl	Infrared	*Hot, penetrating, cleansing, deep heating*
Citrine	Yellow	*Warm, enlivening, cleansing*
Diamond	Indigo	*Stimulating, invigorating, clarifying, antidepressant*

Emerald	Green	*Cold, unifying and solidifying, analgesic*
Ruby	Red	*Heating, drying, energizing, expanding*
Sapphire	Violet	*Tranquillizing, soothing, analgesic, antispasmodic*
Topaz	Blue	*Cool, soft, satisfying, antiseptic*

Combinations

Traditional ayurvedic gem therapy includes the use of certain combinations of gems. Sure enough, these too are effective when supplied electronically. Thus emerald and sapphire make an excellent combination which is cooling, soothing and analgesic. Carnelian and diamond through the chest is a good combination for asthma, to allergically cleanse and energize the struggling lungs. Obesity might be benefited by ruby and diamond, to increase heat and stimulate blood flow, especially if directed to the thyroid to increase metabolism.

Two classical compound mixtures frequently used are IBGO (Indigo-Blue-Green-Orange) or, in other words, diamond-topaz-emerald-carnelian, and the so-called 'Seven Gems' mix which combines all the principal stones except chrysoberyl. These can be used when the picture is complicated, uncertain or simply in cases where generalized light and energy support therapy is needed.

Some conditions, and their suggested gem treatments, are given here and should make the overall principles clear:

Acne	Citrine/Topaz
Alopecia	Sapphire
Anaemia	Ruby
Arthritis	Sapphire/Emerald
Asthma	Carnelian/Diamond
Bronchitis	Citrine/Diamond
Burns	Emerald
Cystitis	Emerald
Conjunctivitis	Carnelian
Constipation	Citrine
Depression	Diamond

Debility	Ruby/Diamond
Diabetes	Diamond/Citrine
Diarrhoea	Emerald
Eczema	Emerald/Sapphire
Epilepsy	Diamond
Gastritis	Emerald
Headache	Sapphire
Insomnia	Sapphire
Irritable bowel	Emerald/Sapphire
Menopause	Carnelian
Migraine	Sapphire
Pain	Sapphire/Emerald
Pleurisy	Topaz
Psoriasis	Sapphire
Rheumatism	Ruby/Sapphire
Sciatica	Sapphire
Shingles	Sapphire/Emerald
Sterility	Diamond
Stomach ulcer	Emerald/Sapphire
Tonsillitis	Topaz
Varicose ulcer	Ruby/Diamond

ELECTRONIC FREQUENCY

There is another dimension completely in this unique Virtual Energy therapy. Because of the introduction of Western electronic technology we are able to add a pulsed frequency to the healing rays. This can enormously influence the power and range of effects. For example, a frequency of 3.3 Hertz (Hz) is identical to the brainwave pattern known as theta, which is associated with trance and dreamlike states (see list of brainwave frequencies, below). If we take emerald and sapphire light and beam it into the skull at 3.3 Hz, the results are quite dramatic. The subject will rapidly descend into a beautiful dreamlike trance, which is very potent at countering stress. We call this *samadhi*, an Indian word meaning 'bliss', which gives a fair description of its subjective result. I use it before all other treatments on my own Caduceus. I argue that all patients are stressed and miserable by virtue of being ill, and this wonderful eased state of mind is a very sound concomitant treatment. The effect lasts up to 24 hours, sometimes longer.

Other useful frequencies are 8 Hz, the Earth's own 'Gaia' resonant frequency, and around 1.5 – 2.5 Hz, which is the lowest band, delta brainwaves. The latter frequency accords with deep unconsciousness and therefore has analgesic potential, rather like an anaesthetic. Combined with soothing emerald it can work wonders for bruised tissue or painful joints.

Logically, diamond would be coupled with 15 – 20 Hz, which is low beta. We never use high beta (above 25 Hz), which is excessively stimulating, since all healing requires calm and ease.

Rhythm	Frequency	State of Consciousness
High beta	above 25 Hz	*Anxiety, panic, anger, psychosis*
Beta	14 – 25 Hz	*Attention focuses on external affairs, 'normal waking'*
Alpha	7.8 – 14 Hz	*Relaxed, attention divided between internal and external matters*
Theta	3.2 – 7.8 Hz	*Dreaming, trance, hypnosis, internal attention*
Delta	01. – 3.2	*Deep sleep, unconsciousness, coma*

As with all advanced technology, the degree of success with the equipment depends considerably on the knowledge and competence of the practitioner. Whereas anyone can get basic results of value, if the use of electronic gem therapy is combined with a good working knowledge of the alternative models, many possibilities open up. For example, eczema is often a symptom of gut overload, especially liver toxicity ('liver anger'). Therefore supporting energies at, say, Gaia frequency to the liver can be an excellent complement to the direct use of soothing emerald light onto the skin.

Carnelian and diamond is an ideal mixture for the circulation and lymph system (8 Hz) and can be used in many ways, for example in the treatment of varicose ulcer or dependant oedema – the latter can be viewed by the layman as an inefficient heart pumping action. But this mixture can create healing pathways at many deeper levels. Thus diamond and carnelian to the spleen area can produce a dramatic benefit for the immune system, resulting in improvement or elimination of many complex allergies. Whale even reports the resolution of two lymphoma cases (malignant condition of lymphoid tissue).

I myself use the mixtures known as VIBGYOR or 'Seven Gems' to the thymus, since this gland is associated with white cell education and maturity and I am deeply involved with the immune system, being known primarily as an allergist. In addition to detox and homeopathic cleansing of the intercellular tissues, this is of great benefit to the chronically ill patient.

Whale's Caduceus equipment has the further refinement of multiple channels. More than one lamp can be rigged and used simultaneously. Thus, for example, the deeply relaxing *samadhi* can be administered at the same time as other specific organ therapy. Or a stimulating mixture at energizing frequencies can be shone into the thymus gland at the same time that soothing emerald and carnelian at theta are used on allergic eczema of the lower leg.

Electronic gem therapy also lends itself very well to being combined with other healing models. Instead of organ or tissue support therapy, excited light can be used to enhance or 'open' chakras.

This is the basis of Whale's claim for enhancing male potency. He has discovered that a series of treatments using ruby light to the base chakra has a powerful stimulating effect and is certainly safer and preferable to modern drug and psychotherapy prescriptions for this commoner-than-supposed condition.

Diamond and topaz to the throat chakra will sometimes produce an immediate change in voice and expression, and 'Seven Gems' to the heart chakra is the nearest thing we have to a treatment for lost love and the pain of separation.

Naturally, this is further support for the validity and existence of chakras since they can be positively influenced in this way, the results becoming unarguably manifest in *this* reality.

Casebook: Female, 45 Years

A woman therapist had torn a muscle in an amateur stage production. The noise of the muscle rupture was so loud it was heard in the second row. She was promptly incapacitated and in great pain.

She came to see me a few days later, limping badly, all other attempts at therapy having failed. I gave her first a routine 20 minutes of *samadhi*, with emerald-sapphire stones at 3.3 Hz. This very aware patient was able to tell me that her pelvis underwent a shift back into the normal energetic position during this stage.

I followed through with about 30 minutes to the injured calf. All pain had now vanished from the affected leg, but now a new pain had appeared in the opposite knee. This was probably due to the stress of limping and bearing all her weight on that side, but the pain had, of necessity, been suppressed.

A further 15 minutes on the uninjured side removed that discomfort too, and the patient walked to her car with no discernible limp. Next day she phoned to say there was only mild discomfort, she was back at work and she was content with just one treatment.

Casebook: Male, 6 Years

This boy had been diagnosed as having disintegrative psychosis, a variety of autism which I have long suspected comes on after vaccination, particularly for measles. My reasoning was as follows: an autistic youngster seems to be very 'out of contact' and 'dreamy'; he (they are usually males) is very introverted into the right brain hemisphere. If we can use the gem therapy to accelerate the left brain and inhibit right-brain activity, we may be able to wake up his logical and reasoning faculties.

Accordingly, I put him on a one-week programme of diamond, citrine and ruby to the left cranial hemisphere and emerald-sapphire to the right brain. I further refined this strategy by using beta (high brain activity) of around 15 Hz to the left side and a retarding and soothing 3.3 Hz to the right hemisphere. I lowered the penetration to minimal wattage in order not to 'cross-over' and inadvertently stimulate the opposite side, or vice versa.

Within days he began vocalizing well and within a month was forming intelligible sentences. For a number of reasons he was unable to continue any further treatments with the Caduceus Lux III, but despite this he continued to make rapid progress. He has learned to use a computer keyboard and happily spends hours amusing himself with electronic games, which of course require considerable left-brain dexterity. His mother reports he has learned to integrate well with his peers. One year later I had a report he is now regraded as mentally normal for schooling purposes.

One of my major plans for the future is to explore this healing route for autism.

BIOLUMANETICS

Nature has the endless capacity to surprise and fascinate us. Biolumanetics, a new science of healing, is just about the most unusual medical application of light in therapy I have heard of. The system was developed by a 62-year-old American engineer called Patrick Richards. In 1983 he designed an instrument called a Luminator™ which balances air temperatures for efficient office energy management. In fact his invention turned out to have a far more important and totally novel application than the one for which it was made.

While testing the unit in an open plan office, Richards found that many people reported unexpected health gains, from reduction of stress and migraine levels to disappearance of low back pain. The big question was – *Why?*

The Luminator™ alters the local environment in three main ways:

1 Temperatures are balanced uniformly throughout (wall-to-wall, floor-to-ceiling).
2 An altered magnetic field is created.
3 The available light in the room is altered from incoherent (light going in many directions) to coherent (polarized into one plane only).

In 1985 Richards discovered by serendipity that light from living cell forms could be imaged in the field of the Luminator™. Late 1985 found him photographing people holding their medications and noting how, as Abrams and Voll had discovered before, that the patient's energy status alters for the better dramatically. In the case of Richards' equipment, a sick person may have a very blurred, indistinct image, but simply by holding an effective medication the person's special photographic image becomes immediately sharp and clear. Logically, if the medication is not suitable, the image remains blurred or becomes even more foggy.

Subsequently, Richards went on to develop a unique and sophisticated method of assessing patients and establishing suitable remedies. He calls his system VRIC (visual reference of image coherence) and it basically entails the use of enhanced photography to measure the vitality and coherence of any life form — human, plant or animal. To make a VRIC assessment image requires a fixed focus Polaroid camera and the Luminator™ as a source. The brightness, intensity and coherence of the light reflected by the patient and captured on the photograph is a precise indication of his or her health and energy status[6]. Therapy would then consist of taking a base image and endeavouring to find a remedy, or more than one remedy, which will make it sharper and brighter, much as the EAV practitioner does by eliminating the ID drop.

Arguably this is a milestone development for practitioners in the field of energetic healing, indeed all therapeutic practice. We can now see objective changes after Reiki, homeopathy, flower essences, shiatsu and colour therapy, to name just a few.

Again, the vital side of the body energy information field is made abundantly clear: the medication need only be put on the floor close to the subject to transmit its signal. No contact is required, but provided it is within the energetic aura the light coherence may change markedly. No smoke, no mirrors! That's about as much 'proof' as we have for you at present of the tenets of energy healing expounded in these pages.

A patient can of course bring his or her own medication for assessment, but VRIC specialists have their own repertoire of preferences and a range of special frequencies called 'Lumanetics' which Richards claims are not affected by Gaia fields. When a suitable therapeutic match is made, the 'vibrational signature' is transferred to an anionic chelate fluid, which is a negatively-charged fluid made in a special field. It is said not only to hold the required therapeutic energy but actually to bind magnetically with toxins and impurities in order to help them be eliminated,[7] though I find statements like this hard to take without some experimental support.

Probably the most exciting potential of all with the VRIC system is in assessing the energy dynamics of interpersonal relationships. The photograph can tell a person if the partner he or she is with is 'right' for them or not. The common complaint 'I feel really drained with that person' can now be expressed in an objective and impersonal way. With a stressful individual standing in close proximity to the subject, the assessment image is blurred, whereas with other neutral companions it remains relatively sharp. It is remarkable to reflect just how radical a change it could bring to our turbulent over-emotional society to be able to assess family, love relationships, professional and personal relationships (in fact any relationship at all) in a clear, precise and *non-judgemental* manner.

On a recent visit to the practice facility of Thrity Engineer, a London-based practitioner of Biolumanetics, I was shown several fascinating examples of family group dynamics. In one instance, a child taking Ritalin for ADD (attention deficit disorder) was quite coherent without the medicine. When his sibling and father stood next to him, he remained fully coherent. But as soon as his mother joined the group, the child's image went incoherent. The surprising course of action was therefore to given the *moth-*

er a remedy, which made the boy coherent again when she held it. The mother was subsequently treated and the boy recovered completely, without any further need of medication.

Thrity also showed me what Richards calls right-and-left-brain-coherence. This is accessed by photographing the patient with the left eye open, right eye closed and then vice versa. An individual will sometimes be incoherent in one modality but not the other.

Casebook: Female, 43 Years

A woman was distressed by the loss of her son some years before. When she held a photograph of the deceased in her right hand (left brain), she remained coherent. But when the photograph was put in her left hand (right brain) she became quite visually incoherent. It is easy to see that she could rationalize her loss (left brain logic) but could not come to terms with the emotions (right brain).

A suitable remedy was chosen photographically and her emotional patterns changed at once to a better and healthier regard for her lost offspring.

Incidentally, I was fascinated to see that even the house-plants which appear in Thrity's photographs would become incoherent along with an incoherent human source nearby. But recovered fully next to a healthy individual!

Biolumanetics claims not to address directly the symptoms of illness. There is nothing to tell the practitioner at what level the bio-energetic disturbance lies, whether energetic, emotional or physical. Thus the approach question is not 'What is causing this incoherence?' but 'What will make this system vital or coherent?'

LASERS

We all know one of the buzzwords for advanced technology is the laser. It is coherent light, produced synthetically; it does not exist in nature, except as ultra weak luminescence (page 51). I have indicated this may be the defining nature of living tissue.

Not surprisingly then, lasers have potential for carrying information into the body; it was merely a matter of time before someone would put this potential to use.

A number of bioenergetic specialists have worked with lasers, giving diverse insights into the BER process along the way. Schimmel has recently brought out a version of the Vega machine which uses a laser probe, instead of the former clumsy blunt-ended probe (the Vega Select). However here I am referring to the practise of shining laser light into acupunture points, or more generally into the energetic aura, carrying therapeutic signals of the kind we have studied along the way in *Virtual Medicine*.

An example of the former is the work of performance scientist Ken West. Ken is American but I met him living and working in the UK. He knew of studies by Prof. Yoshito Mukaino, of Fukuoka University, showing a 20% increase in ball speed of athletes, as a result of checking and balancing acupuncture meridians (surprise!)[8]. Mukaino's work has now become widely accepted and many athletes around the world use his "Meridian Test".

In conjunction with Dr Dane Oosthuizen, Ken has developed a system called "Paradox Medicine" and he's now back in the US (New Mexico) getting great results with it.

Ken deals a lot with various sports injuries, knows the Reckeweg remedies, and has been experimenting with a hand-held laser gun, for both performance enhancement and healing of injuries. He simply shines light through the remedy onto the skin, at suitable sites. For reasons that are not quite clear, this seems to work better if Japanese acupuncture or Jin Shan points are used. These are fewer in number than the Chinese points and, although there is some overlap, are rather different. Ken describes the Japanese points as "deeper" and reverts to Chinese points if the patient is young, old or weak.

Ken's work is also interesting to me in that he has boiled the entire HEEL* repertory of remedies down to about a dozen items. By examining diligently each of the compounded remedies, he found many contained the same substances, grouped in different ways; by using this much narrower range of products, he was able to administer to his patients almost the complete repertory.

Ken has indentified three main groups of remedies: Galium-HEEL® group (drainage), Traumeel® group (immune defense) and Coenzyme compositum® group (metabolic support). Each of these is connected to 3 others, making a list of 12 in all.

[*the full HEEL range, by the way, is reproduced by Biological Homeopathic Industries (BHI) in Albuquerque, New Mexico].

MASTER REMEDY	RELATED REMEDIES
Galium group	Thyroidea comp.
	Cerebrum comp.
	Mucosa comp.
Traumeel group	Echinacea comp.
	Engystol comp.
	Lymphomyosot
Coenzyme comp. group	Ubichinon comp.
	Hepar comp.
	Zeel comp.

However Ken added another remedy which he described as the hand grenade you lob (into the tissues) and cover your ears for the bang! I knew instantly he was talking about HEEL's Glyoxal compositum®.

I myself would add one other super-defense and strengthening remedy and Ken agreed: Discus compositum®, making 14 in all. This sounds like a plug for HEEL, I know, but they *are* good.

Given that laser light is so intense, Ken and I discussed the possibility of overloading the tissues with too much information. In fact this is only theoretical since, if we believe our (Virtual Medicine) model, only those substances the body actually needs will resonate with it. The rest will have no effect (much like a piano will hum or sing with certain notes near it, but will "ignore" the rest of the musical scale).

Ken extended this model usefully, by saying that perhaps the body cycled through levels. On the first round it would take certain remedies or oscillations. Others that were ignored at first, will have an effect later on, as the system dynamics of the living organism change.

He offered a useful tip, anyway, for those practitioners who feel they may be encountering tissue stress, as a result of heavy de-tox-ing: the use of homeopathically potentized vitamin B3 (niacin; don't use niacinamide). This makes sense to me since, as I explained in my last allergy book, niacin is a key precursor to NADH detox path-ways; a strong reducing agent.

CHAPTER 10

GAIA

This is a book about human health and the biological significance of electromagnetism and other energy forces in diagnosis and healing. Quantum potential fields are invoked to explain some of the stranger manifestations which can be observed objectively. But in this chapter we must make the point that we are all subject to much larger energy influences, which are great in magnitude and inescapable by life on Earth. I am referring to the Earth's own energies.

Those of us who care about such things think a lot about the extent to which our lives are influenced by the field phenomena from the 'Earth Mother' or Gaia, as James Lovelock called it[1]. A few years ago it would have been regarded as absurd to consider that the Earth's magnetic field could possibly have an effect on a mammalian species such as humans. Today the only intelligent question, and an important one, is: How could the Earth's electromagnetic energy field possibly *not* have a profound influence on our biology and health?

It is absurd to suppose that this rich and enormous variable energy field has no relevance to our well-being. We may feel we are important from our own limited perspective, but on the bigger scale of things we are quite inconsequential, in orders of magnitude, compared to the Earth's overwhelmingly greater presence. Just because we have hitherto had no awareness of the phenomenon and no satisfactory means of measuring its biological effects does not mean these don't exist. We have been naïve for far too long.

It has become increasingly clear that Gaia is a health issue, as well as an ecological one. Remember Abrams' reflex (where neurologist Albert Abrams noticed a strange dull percussion note when tapping certain areas of his patients' abdomens, which turned up not only in cancer and tuberculosis cases, but even in healthy patients situated in close proximity to cancer or tuberculosis specimens – see Chapter 1). The *big* clue here was the fact that the critical diagnosis could only be made with the patient oriented east—west.

There is a newly-emerged phenomenon we call geopathic stress, meaning that there are certain spots on the Earth which are unhealthy due to distortion of the Earth's field at that point. Many patients will not respond to treatment, particularly any that relies on manipulation of biological energy such as most of the natural therapies, unless any pre-existing geopathic stress is removed.

But the issue is far bigger than this, as we shall see.

THE EARTH'S FIELD

The earth's core is a spinning mass of molten iron. It sets up a huge magnetic field (known variably as the geomagnetic field or magnetosphere), which merges at the poles and spreads out into space for thousands of kilometres. But this field in turn is greatly influenced by an even more powerful energy field: that of the sun. We speak today of 'solar wind', which means the outpourings of charged electrical particles streaming into space with incredible energies, pushing matter before it (there is enough force to propel a rocket up to nearly the speed of light, given time). Most of the force is dissipated into empty regions, but where it meets the magnetic field of a planet, such as the Earth, there are considerable interactions.

On the solar side of the Earth the geomagnetic field is compressed by the pressure of particles and radiation travelling at or near the speed of light. On the far side, the geomagnetic field is thrust far out into space. Certain regions on the sunward side are 'sandwich layers' where high-energy particles are trapped, bouncing around endlessly and forming a kind of cushion. These layers are called the Van Allen belts, after their discoverer. If it were not for the presence of the Van Allen belts, absorbing and damping

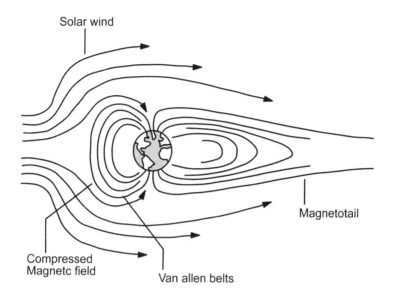

Solar wind

Magnetotail

Compressed
Magnetc field

Van allen belts

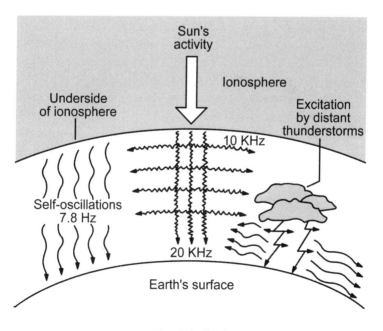

Sun's
activity

Ionosphere

Underside
of ionosphere

Excitation
by distant
thunderstorms

10 KHz

Self-oscillations
7.8 Hz

20 KHz

Earth's surface

The Gaia fields

radiation, life on Earth would be totally unsustainable, except far underground.

It comes as a shock to realize that our friendly sun's rays are so deadly to life. Astronauts can only survive for short periods in space without being shielded, and rocket missions are carefully timed to avoid maximum solar radiation. Outside the Earth's protective magnetosphere humans would be sizzled if they chanced to be caught in a solar storm. I make this point in the hope that it gives a vivid picture of the hostility of the sun's radiation and what we would potentially face down here on the surface, if our protection should fail.

The sun has great power for health and healing, but it would be absurd to think it was not capable of an adverse influence, even at the radiation levels we experience.

ELECTRICAL FIELD

The Earth's magnetosphere does not rotate because the sun's forces grip it. Instead the planetary rock-and-iron ball rotates once every 24 hours within the vast energy shell. On the principle of a dynamo, this generates enormous electrical charges, in the range of billions of watts, even when the sun is quiescent. It is as if we were living inside a cosmically-scaled electrical machine. The dynamo effect also results in ionizing radiation (the deadly radiation of atomic bombs) and extremely low-frequency (ELF) radiation which causes strange and unhealthy biological disturbances.

Any particular spot on the Earth's surface passes through the magnetic field once every 24 hours, from high to low and back again, giving us our basic diurnal variations. It is more important than light levels, and because of it the passage of day can be felt even in total darkness.

Considering the dangerous highly charged natural environment in which we live, it stands to reason that life has evolved very precariously. We could all be snuffed out like the dinosaurs at any moment.

But this also tells us that life here is, for the present, cleverly adapted to this background radiation. Provided the variations are not too large, we can accommodate them.

However, there are times when the sun erupts into extra activity. At these times, the powers unleashed are almost unimaginable to us. The intensity of the solar wind rises and the dangers from the emissions are obviously increased many-fold. The beautiful aurorae or flickering coloured sheets of light in the polar night skies are one of the relatively fortunate consequences. More problematical is the widespread disruption of computers, navigational equipment and telecommunications apparatus.

Fortunately this is not too common an occurrence. But it is hardly surprising, in view of the brain's electrical properties, that at these times people's behaviour may become disturbed. It isn't common knowledge, but there is a marked rise in psychiatric hospital admissions at times of peak sunspot activity. This statistic alone makes it clear that the sun's rays can be bad for us and that Gaia isn't all sweetness and light.

MAGNETIC REVERSALS

The truth is, we have survived on Earth partly because of and partly despite the sun's influence. There are worrying events in the past which may dent the 'friendly goddess' Gaia image. Every once in a while the Earth's magnetic field undergoes a tremendous upheaval and reverses itself; north pole to south and vice versa. Typically these transformations have taken around 10,000 years, which might seem a long time to a human but is a mere blink of an eye in geological terms.

Nobody knows why these cataclysmic reversals take place, but one thing is very clear: they are deadly to life, leading to widespread extinction of species, particularly animal life. This is probably because the magnetosphere dies away during the transition and the protective fields such as the Van Allen belts cease to shield the planetary surface from the ferocity of the sun's radiation.

As an aside, these mass die-offs make nonsense out of Darwinian evolution, though some scientists have tried to explain the discrepancies of Darwin's theories by inventing 'punctuated equilibrium'. By this contrivance the theory of a slow, tortured evolution is kept alive. Once Vitalism (see Chapter 1) is understood and embraced, these crutches to mechanistically-conceived life will prove unnecessary.

Is this phenomenon of reversal relevant to us? Well, we cannot predict – as we can with the mathematical probability that the next major meteorite impact is actually long overdue – when the next magnetic field reversal will take place. Contemporary measurements tell us that the intensity of the Earth's field has been on the wane for several decades. But Robert Becker writes that this is largely an academic matter: we have produced far more than the equivalent of a magnetic field reversal by virtue of the magnetic outpourings that Man himself has created.[2] Becker calls it electro-pollution. We have created our own dangerous environment and it is already having a health impact.

ARTIFICIAL RADIATION

Most people overlook the fact that microwaves and radio waves are part of the electromagnetic spectrum, parts of which are deadly (x-rays, alpha rays and gamma rays). The medical profession was caught off-guard too, and for a time microwave heating of the tissues (diathermy) was considered an excellent treatment for a wide variety of conditions. Just what microwaves are capable of is seen clearly by the effect on a good steak.

But just because radio waves carry our favourite television programmes and the sound of audience laughter does not mean they are safe. In fact we are now exposed to a combined radiation exposure from all sources which exceeds a million-fold the natural background radiation in which we evolved as a species.

As you will have gathered, we are biological beings which exist as an energy cloud, in the presence of a physical body (proven). This makes us very vulnerable to the damaging effects from extraneous electromagnetic energy fields. We should be concerned about how to protect ourselves from these hostile forces. Geopathic stress, the term we now use, goes beyond the way in which Gaia's own energies can influence us and refers also to the influence of man-made electromagnetic radiations, from computer VDUs, microwave ovens, TV screens, cell phones and so on. Many of us spend hours a day at the personal computer and unless you have an LCD screen that means a considerable dose of electromagnetic radiation including, on some models, soft x-rays. The doses may be small but are cumulative.

Try this revealing test

Try this simple test with your cell phone, if you use one. Put it into the microwave oven, close the door and dial it. If the phone rings (and it will!) the shielding on your microwave oven is shown to be worthless and you should get rid of it, for safety's sake. If microwaves can get IN, microwaves can get OUT.

Probably the biggest microwave hazard today is the cell phone and the accompanying base towers. The communications industry is now becoming so sneaky, they are disguising masts as palm trees, water towers and other inconspicuous objects, so that they are fast becoming a part of our general landscape.

One patient in the San Francisco Bay area was constantly sick. She moved apartments, feeling sure the cause was environmental, and felt slightly better for a time. But as the problem got worse, she investigated and found that the first apartment had *over 1500 transmitting antennas within a 10-block radius*. The second apartment had 941 within 10 blocks. She was OK for about a year and a half before the symptoms again became pronounced.

She now believes, in retrospect, that it was when this later apartment complex struck a deal with Ygnition to install wireless antennas throughout the complex to provide all the tenants with a wireless Internet service that she began having symptoms once more. The last straw was a new neighbor who moved in next door and put a wireless router on the other side of the wall from her bed. At this stage she would wake up and have to hold on to the wall, she felt so dizzy!

If you want to know how many antennas are transmitting near you, visit: http://www.antennasearch.com, type in your address.

PROTECTIVE DEVICES?

There are many devices on the market now which it is claimed will protect us from cell phone radiation. Some are no more than little absorbent pads which stick to your phone or its battery. Others are pouches with Faradic cage-type screening.

Certainly the best advice I can offer is avoid cell phones as much as is humanly possible. I despair of those I see walking around or driving with a phone endlessly slapped to their temples. The dangers are not in question; only the scruples of the phone industry are questionable. Never hold one to your head for more than a few moments. Get an ear piece.

However, there is still a problem; the cord to the ear piece acts as an antenna and may actually intensify the radiation to which you are exposed and direct it to your head. This is partly solved by attaching a small hematite bead to the cable, which impedes the passage of microwave pulses.

But safer by far is to use an earpiece which is connected only via a terminal section of air tube. The loudspeaker is several inches from the earpiece and the sounds are delivered from there along the air tube (rather like a doctor's stethoscope). Thus no electromagnetic fields are relayed to the head. Beyond that I can offer little positive.

I am sure that we are yet to inherit a blizzard of cases damaged by their addictive use of this insidious device. The real question that keeps going round in my mind is not so much "Why do they do it?" but actually "What did people do before cell phones?" Were they really so empty-headed as to be constantly bored or to feel the need of conversation in order to recognize their own worth?

I have repeatedly referred to the obvious biological dangers of electromagnetic fields. Magnetic fields above 3 milligauss are thought to be dangerous. But electrical fields too

The original safety standard for radiation dosage of the microwave type was set at $100mW/cm^2$, which was based on the dose required to produce body heating. This was soon dropped to $10mW/cm^2$ but there it has stuck and the fallacy has arisen that this is a scientifically-judged figure.

DIRTY ELECTRICITY

Roger Coghill, research scientist, consultant and author of *Something in the Air*, tells me that current thinking is that electrical fields are probably more critical than magnetic flux, as was for-

merly thought. He recommends a safe level of 50 nanoTesla (nT).
Danger is certainly present beyond 250 nT. (A nanoTesla is about
10 volts per square metre). As Coghill points out, someone who
spends most of his or her time in a typical home with levels of,
say, 200–250 nanoTesla may actually receive more radiation in a
year than someone who lives in a 'safe' house but is exposed to
occasional doses of thousands or even tens of thousands of nano-
Tesla.[5]

My big concern today however is what has become termed
"dirty electricity". You would be right to expect that the utility
company mains supply is a nice "clean" 60 Hz. This itself is biological stressful enough—but survivable.

However, the typical supply is far from clean. It contains many
large surges or spikes, typically in the 10 kHz - 50 kHz radio frequency (RF) range. These are introduced by numerous electrical
devices, which may not even be in your home but from a neigh-
bour or even an industrial facility somewhere nearby. Dimmer
switches, plasma screens, fluorescent lights and loose wire connections around the home are common sources of this problem.

These sudden surges, or "transients" as they are known in the
trade, are extremely damaging to computers and sensitive electronic equipment: you may even have a surge protector already
fitted to your computer input supply. Motors and transformers
will burn out. Without this protection, equipment would soon be
rendered non-functional.

Yet nobody seems to care so much about this same effect on
humans. Yet I have found this to be a common unsuspected cause
of all kinds of health ills, from headaches to chronic fatigue and
even cancer clusters.

SPILLAGE

Another major health hazard has emerged with the recognition that utility companies are cheating. They are permitted to
"dump" a certain amount of current to earth but in fact they are
returning as much as 70% of their neutral current to ground. It
makes its way back to the power station any way it can and may
in fact travel miles of detour, visit *your* home and others nearby,

before completing its circuit. Electricity will follow the path of least resistance (Ohm's Law) and NOT necessarily the shortest distance from A to B. What's more electricity is not bound to follow only one path (Kirchoff's Law).

The upshot of this is that any building can become dangerously charged. If you stand with barefeet on a tile floor and touch a metal pan to the tap, you may receive a very significant charge (up to 80 microamps: enough to trigger heart fibrillation).

Moreover it makes a lunacy of wiring your household appliances with a ground to earth, such as a water pipe, *because this may be bringing current into your house and not conducting it away safely, as it is supposed to do.*

Get your home checked by someone with a sensitive meter and the competence to tell you what is really happening (do NOT ask the utility company to make tests; they lie).

WHAT YOU CAN DO

If you are concerned and would like to reduce your radiation exposure levels, you can help yourself quite a lot.

- Remove all unnecessary electrical devices from your bedroom, such as electric alarm clocks, radios and tea-makers.
- Get rid of electric blankets permanently. Forget about water beds; these create and hold a substantial field.
- Avoid electrical equipment as much as possible but especially don't group it near where someone sits or sleeps.
- You can have an EMF (electromotive force) demand switch fitted to your domestic supply which will turn off the mains at night but continue to supply the refrigerator and freezer (thus keeping you electricity-free for at least 8 hours a day.
- Stay at least 3 metres from your television screen and do not allow children to sit up close to it.
- If you have a mobile phone, keep the phone as far away from your brain as possible and fit a proper shield or use the alternatives I have suggested.
- Fit damping filters to prevent "dirty electricity" spikes. I recommend the Stetzer-Graham units, which can be obtained from: www.stetzerelectric.com

- If you use a computer or VDU, at home or at work, try to place it as far from your body as possible. Insist on a protective screen. Make sure you are not contaminated by someone else's equipment, either nearby or in the next room (soft x-rays and microwaves can travel through walls unhindered).
- Avoid precautionary or 'routine' medical and dental x-rays for check-up purposes. Women of childbearing years should have x-rays only in the 10 days following menstruation. Though this is now in dispute, it is better to play safe. Allow no x-rays whatever if you are trying to conceive. Children should never be x-rayed, except in a dire emergency.

Caution

Do not attempt any kind of screening or Faradic cage for protection, using meshes, metal plates or wires. *You could make things worse by inadvertently focusing or intensifying the electromagnetic fields.*

If you want to measure the ambient levels of radiation exposure, consider one of the simple field meters which are available on the Internet. You can get gauss meters (magnetic fields) and electrical field meters separately. Roger Coghill manufactures and sells a hand-held device called a *Field Mouse* which is designed to warn of levels over 200 nT or 25 V/m^2 (available from Coghill Research Laboratories).

Stetzer-Graham produce a special meter to measure transient mains spikes. It is available from www.stetzerelectric.com

SCHUMANN WAVES

One aspect of Earth's radiation which has only recently attracted attention as a health issue is the Schumann wave effect. The Earth's atmosphere, between the underside of the ionosphere and the surface (especially the salt oceans) forms what scientists call a resonating cavity magnetometer. Due to excitation by the Earth's own magnetism, sunspots and lightning storms, this cavity emits a transverse resonating waveband that we call Schumann waves, after the man who discovered them in the 1940s.

The actual frequency varies according to the height of the ionosphere and large-scale weather patterns, but is generally in the 8—10 Hertz range. I feel sure it is no coincidence that this frequency is virtually identical with that of the hippocampus of mammalian species.

What is worrying is that modern cities have very low levels of Schumann waves, as most of these waves are absorbed by the vast masses of concrete and metal buildings. The gradual lowering of the land water table has also added to the deficiency.

This must have severe and unavoidable health consequences for city dwellers. The loss of health-giving Schumann waves could be a contributory factor in 'sick building syndrome'. However, caution is needed. Simply supplying Schumann waves carries with it the very distinct danger of increased platelet aggregation (blood clotting); this in turn is a known risk factor in heart disease and strokes.

The key to this further complication seems to be 'plasma waves'. These are interactions between the Earth's magnetic field and mineral elements within the lithosphere (Earth's crust). The strength of the waves generated is very small, even by the standards of the Gaia fields, but what seems to be important is a resonance effect between the Earth's minerals and the same elements within living forms, especially the blood.[6]

At first sight it might appear that the oscillations from the electron shells of very many elements at once would simply create 'noise'. However, according to new theories, electron plasma waves have precise frequencies in the extremely low frequency (ELF) band (which, as I keep repeating, has a powerful biological impact). Trace minerals are present in very tiny amounts as constituents of vitamins, enzymes and hormones. Resonant frequencies from the Earth in these critical bands could have an enormous effect on these body chemical mediators, through the mechanism of cyclotron resonance, which I explained in the first chapter.

If this is correct then we do seem to be, literally, children of Gaia and will have difficulty adjusting to other worlds that we may in time visit.

THE GRIDS

As I reported in my book *The Allergy Handbook*, skilled dowsers have been able to find definite geometric grids which cross and re-cross the Earth's surface.[7] I refer here to the Curry Grid and the Hartman Net (both named after the doctors who discovered them). I am *not* here including ley lines.

I have great confidence in the ability of certain dowsers and therefore accept the presence of these grids. Far too many people can find them. I myself have felt the rods kick when I was shown what to do by the great Kathe Bachler. However, I have always been troubled by the oddity of such geometric straightness or rigidity being imposed upon the natural organic order of things. I have since come across a model which may help us to gain more insight into this possibility.

It comes from an experiment carried out by pupils of Buckminster Fuller. A balloon submerged in coloured fluid and subject to vibration revealed geometric patterns where the dye had broken up into intersecting straight lines over the surface of the sphere. The classic icosahedron of the geodesic dome developed by Fuller came from this observation. It is truly a Gaia design. From this experiment it does seem that there are inherent energy formations on the surface of a sphere which follow straight lines (though not, of course, truly straight but bent to the shape of the sphere).

I was interested to learn that Polynesian sailors were able to navigate by following bands of 'light' under the ocean. Only a fool would now scoff at this idea. Perhaps the Australian aboriginal dream lines are also in some way connected with this surface grid phenomenon.

I don't want to wander off into the realms of so-called Earth mysteries, ley lines, ancient temple sites and so on, though I can't exclude the possibility that they may be aspects of the same thing. I am merely making the point that there is a natural scientific validity in the existence of electromagnetic grids and patterns over the Earth's surface, and wish to imply the logical corollary that these must perforce have a health impact, for good or ill.

Such energy networks will also form a background of interference with the biological energy signals which can be detected by the equipment you have been reading about in this book.

RADIOACTIVITY

One of the most frightening and significant stressors of the human body arising in modern times is ionizing radiation pollution. It is appropriate to include this in a review of Gaia since, initially, radon seepage from rock such as granite or (more rarely) uranium was our only source of this deadly energy. Nowadays humanity produces such huge quantities of radioactivity that we are truly soiling our own nest and facing dire consequences.

It is an irony that radiation has saved the lives of many thousands of people, yet it is deadly to cells and all living tissue. Radiotherapy is now such a key feature of anti-cancer therapies that one may be forgiven for losing sight of the fact that it actually *causes* cancer. X-rays are so dangerous that mass radiography programmes had to be discontinued; it was concluded that screening for breast cancer was actually causing 5 per cent more cancers than it was detecting!

'Ionizing' radiation means that which harms us by causing alterations in the electrical status of the atoms and molecules of our body substances by wrecking the normal electrical bonding. The resulting charged particles are highly aggressive and can damage and even kill tissues when released. The extent of the damage depends on the dose, and herein is one of the major problems with this particular hazard, which is that doses are cumulative for life. That means all the radiation you have ever been faced with is added together in a running total. It does not 'wear off'.

In sufficient doses (by convention we speak as if it were a drug or medicine!) it causes radiation sickness, which is characterized by severe tissue damage, leading to loss of hair, loss of intestinal mucosa and severe disruption of the blood-forming tissues. The latter is particularly important, since it means the possibility of both anaemia and white cell (leukocyte) failure. Loss of viable leukocytes means the body is unable to defend itself from pathogens or cancerous invasion. Death is the usual outcome of severe radiation sickness. There is little that can be done to treat it. Those who survive often go on to develop cancer, leukaemia and, as we saw from Hiroshima and Nagasaki, genetic malformations.

Unfortunately, there is no 'standard' disease befalling an individual who has passed the safe quota for radiation. The effects show up simply as an increase in existing pathological conditions. This allows a great deal of official fudging about the true dangers of living near nuclear plants and 'hot' military installations.

By its very nature, the effects of chronic insidious exposure to ionizing radiation goes largely undetected, since we have no biological sensors with which to measure it. It is only when recognized polluters see fit to install monitoring equipment that we may know what is actually happening to our environment and the extent of the threat to our health. Spectacular melt-downs such as that at Chernobyl and the narrowly-averted Three Mile Island disaster may be the stuff we all fear; but there is good reason to believe that far more people are killed by radiation annually, without realizing it, than ever died in all the disasters put together. Again, official secrecy is keeping us in the dark, as if it were a government's right to deceive and dissemble to its people.

Yet leaks do occur. Such releases are not confined to nuclear reactors or weaponry, but take place at all stages of processing, from mining to the disposal of waste. Once in the environment, radioactive elements are concentrated in the food chain. We may be exposed to Caesium 137 in fish stocks up to 1,000 times the normal level; iodine sources are suspect since Chernobyl and, as we all know, strontium 90 has been a dangerous polluter of milk supplies since nuclear testing began in the 1960s.

The trouble is, most of these substances have a very long half-life. For strontium it is only 50 years, but plutonium 239 remains dangerously radioactive for 250,000 years.

CRYSTALS

Finally, to sweeten the note, it is right to take a look at crystals in the context of Gaia. Thus we come back to holism instead of hazards. There is a large and flourishing healing movement using the properties of crystals to improve body energy.[9] The ordered structure of crystals has a constant, coherent and reproducible energy vibration. Crystals can be used to transmit, receive, amplify, modulate (transform) or ground (earth) energies. In fact, society as we know it could not exist without these properties of crystals; they are used in radio, television, computers and other electronic devices. The laser relies absolutely on the coherent intense light propagated by ruby.

Crystals can also store energy. If you hit a crystal with a mallet it will give off a brief flash of visible light; the so-called piezoelectric effect of rock crystal. Earth crust pressures do this on natural rock, as I explain in *The Allergy Handbook*, and this may be the source of many strange 'UFO' effects, especially in mountain zones, such as the Andes, where many strange lights are to be seen.[10]

If you consider that you are no more than flesh and blood, then you might reject the idea that crystals can affect you in any way. But if you have been following the main thread of this book and accept that we are a composite 'energy being' then you will readily understand it is quite obvious that crystals can influence our 'aura'. If you put a coherent crystalline structure in your body energetic field, it is bound to change it in some way; and if you are very sensitive you may even feel this.

Amethyst is known as a *receiver*. It was used in crystal radio sets. Popes and Bishops have traditionally worn amethyst rings to receive messages 'from above'. Rose quartz was also used in the days of crystal radio, but as a transmitter. Tourmaline is an amplifier, aquamarine a tuner and carnelian a grounder. Amazonite is said to open the higher psychic centres. I didn't know of this property when I once carried some in my pocket and had the strangest other-worldly sensations, until I realized what it was and removed it.

If you use a computer a great deal, you might like to introduce a large crystal next to it to absorb some of the radiation. Smoky quartz is said to be best. Try it if you are prepared to believe this section!

CHAPTER 11

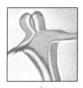

STAR TREK MEDICINE IS HERE... NOW!

As I said in the first edition of Virtual Medicine, a pocket-sized device to defibrillate hearts, rapidly heal sports injuries, strokes, angina, back pains and irritable bowel disease (as well as pre-menstrual tension and post-surgical complications) sounds like a large claim. Yet by the late 1990s this was what was being asserted for a family of medical devices called the SCENAR. S.C.E.N.A.R. is an acronym for self controlled energo-neuro-adaptive regulation (you may also search SKENAR on the Net, since some people spell it that way, but which makes nonsense of the acronym).

There were very few diseases, it was said, that these devices could not treat and often cure, cancer being one of them, though it may be used for painful malignant conditions, avoiding stimulating the tumour itself.

Having obtained and experimented with one, I was very impressed and enthusiastically gave it my support. This new system is a revolutionary approach which again combines the technology of orthodox Western medical practise with ancient knowledge of the East.

The promise of a small hand-held device that seemed capable of curing most illnesses such as was portrayed in the cult 1970s TV series 'Star Trek' had in less than twenty years almost become a reality. I am pleased and amused that my book launched the phrase "Star Trek Medicine" and it has now passed into wide usage.

I remain satisfied that this is a major new advance but I have become aware that there have been outrageous claims, lies told and ugly politics surfaced. Suppliers and teachers of the method vie with one another economically and are not beyond attempting to trash each others' reputation. One supplier is even reputed to be in league with the Russian mafia and other dealers claim to have been threatened. Greed has surfaced in a big way and there are many individuals and companies involved the "boom" who have little holistic health skill or experience.

I have cynically posted two typical threads of development below. You may hear more; believe what you will! When I spoke to one of the Russian developers on their first UK visit, he even muttered something about the origin of the instrument being the deliberate creation of pain. It sounded rather dark and sinister, given the murky political background of 20th century Russian science.

Background story number one

The original inventor of the Scenar is said to be A.A.Karasev an electronics engineer back in 1973 who made one for himself after some of his family members died and the conventional medicine of the day could not help[1].

Karasev later worked for the Russian Cosmonaut program and showed his invention to his superiors who were very interested, so much so that a team was set up with funding to develop the idea further.

When the Soviet Union decided to send cosmonauts into orbit for prolonged periods, it was clear that they needed to have a means of treating any illnesses that could befall them. Unlike the American system, there were no convenient re-usable shuttles to bring an ailing cosmonaut back to Earth, should the need have arisen. The possibility of incapacitating disease was a major worry.

The pharmaceutical approach was not tenable, bearing in mind the rigorous weight and space limitations and the fact that drug-oriented medicine is based on the principle of one substance for each (potential) condition. Even a very modest pharmaceutical range would be weighty. Also, an environment where recycling of water is such an essential feature, any drug entering the water circulation system would persist, passing through fellow cosmonauts many times.

This was when the Russian space program was being watched by the rest of the world and maintaining national prestige was of paramount concern to the Soviet government. It was essential to come up with something radically new. It had to be light, easy to use and, of course, really effective.

Bioresonance technology was the only extant medical paradigm capable of delivering these stringent requirements. By expanding on the theoretical work of P K Anokhin[2], particularly in connection with non-anatomical "functional systems", the team developed elegant new physiological models, which led to the current range of electronic interactive devices.

Ironically, no SCENAR device has been used in space to date. There were delays caused by the authorities insisting on a water-proofing process. Before this matter was resolved, funds were suddenly stopped at the time of perestroika, the so-called space race was called off and the team disbanded. The US began working on combined space projects with the Russians and this introduced the capability of evacuating sick cosmonauts on the shuttle, which meant there was no further need of on-board therapy.

The end of the communist era led to a cessation of funding but some of the members of the team decided to continue and formed the OKB Ritm company in 1983. Names you repeatedly come across are A.N.Revenko, Y.Grinberg, and Y.Gorfinkel as well as Karasev. They managed to get approval in 1986 from the Russian Ministry of Health for the device to be used in health clinics.

Background story number two

The SCENAR devices arose from a study of an Eastern therapy know as 'zonal contact massage'. The intention had been to develop some way of altering the pressure of the massage, according to skin response (readers will recall that in chapter 3 I described how the dialectric potential of collagen tissue is stimulated by pressure). Equipment was developed to tap magnetic effects from the skin and use these to modulate changes in pressure of the massage. A team of scientists, including five research doctors, was involved in the original studies, based in Sochi and Krasnodar.

The establishment of a biofeedback mechanism led to the creation of a device whose output would depend on skin energetic response. The term SCENAR was born. It is yet another brilliant marriage of Western electronic technology and Eastern energetic healing skills.

The aim is to stimulate the body's own endogenous energies to effect the cure, using as a mediator the brain's own internal pharmacy of neuropeptides. This allows the body its own choice of healing ingredients. Through biofeedback a dialogue is formed between the tissues and the instrument, each new signal evolves as a new output. No two consecutive signals from the device are the same. This allows the treatment to be truly dynamic, adjusting for changes in state of the body through time and in different physiological conditions.

Certainly, when you learn the SCENAR properly, you will be impressed that it overlaps well with acupuncture and zonal therapies. You can stimulate acupuncture points and work on meridians. Perhaps this, really, is the true story.

WHAT ACTUALLY HAPPENS?

The Russians make a great deal out of the chemical model and the "on-board" natural pharmacy of the brain. Stimulating the nerve pathways externally with the SCENAR feeds back to the brain and causes the release of case-suitable neuropeptides. The operator does not have to know what these chemical compounds are; just leave it to Nature to select what is best.

Whereas it is nice for some to have the credibility-factor of invoking reticulo-endothelial pathways and neuropeptides, I have never seen any hard evidence adduced for this often-repeated claim.

I think what is much more important and tends to be glossed over is that the SCENAR is an electronic energy healing device. It belongs firmly in the bioresonance model referred to in chapter 6. I discussed this at length with Professor Ravenko and his colleagues at the first launch in Europe (Marlow, 1999) and that is what he propounded.

Liken it, if you will, to throwing a grenade into the enemy bunker. Fixed energies, we know, are the pathological ones. Anything which disrupts these will lead to a re-alignment and transformation to something healthier. Thus strongly overwriting fixed energy patterns with the SCENAR will move things out of status quo and the rest is done by Nature herself.

I brought Morrell and Rache into the conversation (see chapter 6) and Rovenko was indignant that the real founder of bioresonance was Alexander Gurwitsch, whose discovery of ultraweak photon emission from the living systems I described on page 51. This gave rise to biophotonics, showing that light (electromagnetic radiation) was the principle means of communication between cells. You will hear me remark through and through this book that the Russians are much more open to broad-minded and revolutionary concepts than their Western counterparts.

Gurwitsch, incidentally, was also a founder of morphogenetic field theory, long before Rupert Sheldrake made this model popular (page 30).

OPERATION

The impressive technology, though dogged initially by Russian low build-quality, allows modulation of wave forms, frequencies, pulses, damping and intensity, as well as the current or "force" settings. One general mode allows the operator to choose the signal qualities; the other is adapted from the body's own energies, which are altered to a pre-set algorithm and returned to the tissues. I explain this to patients as being rather like two radio programs: on one channel the DJ chooses all the tunes; the other is rather like a request program and incoming calls dictate what is broadcast.

Essentially, SCENAR is using the patient's own endogenous signals on a cybernetic feedback basis, scanning and re-transmitting many times a second. As described to me, the device 'evolves' a new signal pattern for the disordered tissues, the machine literally entering into an information dialogue with the body. New frequencies and energy patterns are established, which in turn become fresh input signals, to be further modified, and so on. This output-equals-new-input is much the way that fractals are generated and thus, biologically-speaking, we seem to be on good ground here.

A word of warning, if you get involved: the Russian fashion is to turn up the current and zap the patient; a crude "Give 'em their money's worth" attitude. This does not truly accord with the principles of energy medicine, which is that it is not the quantity of energy but its nurturing quality that counts. The more-is-better approach is what dogs conventional medicine and so often makes it dangerous. Remember Robert Becker's warning from chapter 2, to beware high energy transfer systems, which overreach the body's own endogenous levels of energy. The capability for causing damage is without question.

Casebook: Male, 69 years:

This patient was a gardener with suppurating osteomyelitis of the foot which could not be controlled. He was scheduled for an amputation of the lower leg in four days time, largely because of the intractable pain. At the last moment a British SCENAR practitioner was called into attempt a treatment. The device was used bi-laterally for around 30 minutes on the first day.

Next day, the leg was pain-free for the first time in eight months. Later that day another 30-minute treatment was given. By next morning the recovery was so dramatic the amputation was called off. A third treatment was given and seven days after the first SCENAR this man was back at work, digging in the garden. His leg has completely recovered.

CLINICAL ASPECTS

No pain is felt but the patient is usually aware of a tingling sensation while it works and some people are very uncomfortable with this. The practitioner seeks for what the Russians term asymmetry, meaning something different about the tissue characteristics in the vicinity.

There are five main criteria:
- colour difference (reddening or pallor)
- sensation (numbness or hyper-aesthesia)
- 'stickiness' in which the machine drags with a magnet like quality as it is drawn over certain tracts of the skin
- sound changes (the machine begins to chatter electronically when it hits the right zone)
- Numerical display readings alter

Even though it may not coincide with the obvious area of symptoms or pathology, the important point is to treat the asymmetry. For reasons we do not fully understand, when this is eliminated, recovery will rapidly follow.

There are few contra-indications, notably heart pacemakers and, after 20 years, a remarkable absence of negative side-effects. One of the complications of therapy, however, is that the instrument battery can (and does) pick up energies from the previous patient and can transfer them adversely to a subsequent person.

Also it is unwise to treat a tumour or work in the region of a known tumour. The energy modifications are random, as explained, and could have an unfortunate consequence. However the SCENAR is good for revitalizing the sagging energies of a seriously ill cancer case and that has tremendous healing value. Ultimately, as Lakhovsky told us, cancer is a "battle of radiations" and the stronger the body's own energies, the better.

WHERE TO GET THE DEVICES

The OKB Ritm company still produces several models using names such as Scenar 97, Scenar NT, Scenar 2003, Autoscenar, Kosmed and, lately, the SCENAR Pro. (http://www.scenar.com.ru/index_eng.html) They have a branch office in the Netherlands. (http://www.ritmedic.com/home.html)

At the risk of offending other manufacturers I can say objectively that the Ritm models are the best built SCENARs, the best performing, with the European CE approval mark and the models with the best training and after service, thanks largely to Jan de Jong of the Dutch suppliers/manufacturers. The official US importers are Pacific Health Options (ironically in Vancouver, Canada) and they have only models, to my knowledge, which have official FDA clearance (for sports injuries and pain relief).

Karasev decided to go his own way in 1990 and set up the LET Medical company which produces a range of models under the Scenar and Cosmodic brands. (http://www.scenar.ru/en/)

The Rema company in Belorussia started producing Prologue and Enart models in 1993. (http://rema.by/) Check out their English powerpoint presentation where it says 'english version' (http://rema.by/?module=about)

CCC Invet is a reseller of several of the above companies products and has an English website. (http://www.invet.net/32/e/about_e.shtml)

Another company RTS ART was set up in 1995 and now trades as Denas MS producing the Denas and DiaDens models. (http://www.denascorp.ru/) They have many resellers some with English websites.

The Pervade Wave company in Hong Kong has a regional (Asia) license to produce the Space Healer model. These are sold in HK (http://www.naturalhealing.com.hk/spacehealer.php) and in Australia (http://www.enlightenedtherapies.com/index.htm)

There is also supposed to be a US-made model the Inter X 5000 from NRG (Neuro Research Group) but it is taking a very long time to come to fruition, if it ever does. (http://www.inter-x5000.com/)

Note that I do not support any of this rash of providers, since it is beyond my ability to vouch for the technical performance of each device or the integrity of each of the companies or individuals concerned.

IT STARTS TO FALL APART!

It seems that Ritm was originally happy to licence the SCENAR idea to other companies, but then when they started to make their own variants disputes arose as to who could use the brand name SCENAR and whose model was better etc. Hence there is quite a lot of mudslinging you have read past.

Most of the companies originally targeted the health care market with expensive products although there are now some cheaper home-use models with reduced features. They also tended to sell training courses to their customers and provided little written documentation.

The exception seems to be the Denas company which decided to go down the network marketing route with large numbers of resellers and reasonable prices. They have four current models including a Euro Denas one with CE certification and an English version of their printed 240 page Denas Therapy Manual and its accompanying 2 hour video, although the English translation could be much improved. Their latest model the Diadens-DT even includes two electro acupuncture modes. This gives it Voll's EAV capabilities, which we met in chapter 4 (http://www.scott-mumby-scenar.com/).

There is now also a PC-compatible model, which will supply a printout suitable to give the patient and file a copy in his or her records for reference.

You can download a good 172 page English manual from Transformation Technologies website. (http://www.braintuner.com/skenar.htm). It is not stated where this manual came from but the preface is signed Sergey Solomko and he is the owner of the Invet company.

I also discovered that there is a wealth of Scenar related information on the internet but unsurprisingly mostly in Russian. However you can use the free online translation engine World-Lingo.

http://www.worldlingo.com/en/products_services/worldlingo_translator.html)

My own take on this is that every home should have one of these devices in the medicine cupboard. The simple "home models" require very little knowledge to use and, although they lack the sophistication of the more elaborate devices, will be very useful for sudden toothaches, sore throats, minor physical injuries and fevers. It has even helped MS sufferers and restored some degree of muscular function and strength.

THE HEALING SHOCK OF CRISIS

One of the reasons I am confident that the SCENAR is more an energy healing device than a neuro-physiological one is the characteristic way that a so-called "healing crisis" or past shock may come to the surface.

It is not uncommon while treating some chronic condition for the body to suddenly erupt in the manifestation of some old but clearly discernable disease. The patient seems to be carried back years in time and experience a cleansing and revival by re-experiencing the former condition. The ensuing illness can be severe and shocking to the patient but the recovery more than justifies the process.

This goes to the very heart of the virtual medicine healing model I have described all through these pages, where an old pathological energy "imprint" is attached to the body and when this is dislodged it will fade and vanish. Unfortunately, sometimes it may induce a temporary reversion to the disease of old, as I described under Hering's Law in page 117. Very likely in these cases the proper natural process of resolution has been interrupted by antibiotics or some other drug intervention which left the acute illness suspended, only to emerge years later as a chronic disease or condition.

Operating with other modalities

One of the appealing aspects of the SCENAR I have found is the easy interaction with other healing modalities. For examples, SCENAR stimulation can be applied to acupuncture points. The results may enhance both modalities.

Thus pressure on the point Colon #4 at the base of the thumb can bring deeply buried old emotions to the surface and a resolution. On one occasion I applied a SCENAR to my own lung #7 and that brought a burst of tears; this is also a notorious emotional point! We have the expression "getting it off one's chest" for emotional release, don't we?

Other points worth considering are:
• Bladder #47 -- helps to release repressed fear and encourages feelings of strength resolution.

- Kidney #6 -- this point may be used for stage fright or fears about any performance.
- Triple Heater #15 -- this point helps relax nervous tension associated with worry.
- Stomach # 36 -- helps to reduce anxiety by strengthening the entire energetic and physical body.

SCENARs also adapt very well with the auriculo-acupuncture method of Nogier, described on pages 49- 50.

SCENARs can be skillfully combined with knowledge of myofascial triggers points. These are described as hyperirritable spots in skeletal muscle that are often palpable as nodules in taut bands of muscle fibers. These are said to be the origin of a great deal of soft-tissue pain. The trigger point may not be where the pain is felt (referred pain) so it took a little time for this phenomenon to come to light.

The trigger point concept still remains unknown to most doctors and is not generally taught in medical school curricula. The most recent definitive work is by Janet G. Travell and David Simons (*The Trigger Point Manual*)[3]. Travell was so successful at treating John F. Kennedy's back pain that she became the first female Personal Physician to the President.

Because of this versatility the SCENAR is exceptional for sports injuries and has kept many a professional athlete on the field, instead of being laid up in bed.

In fact for pain relief, it is quite exceptional. I have seen it dispel severe biliary colic, toothache and the pain of a fracture through the ankle in a matter of minutes (biliary colic—gallstones—is one of medicine's two worst pains; the other is a kidney stone).

COSMETICS AND EYE BENEFITS

One of the surprising additional benefits of the SCENAR has been its use as a cosmetic device. It is excellent for toning muscles and can thus be used to reverse some of the facial damage of aging, removing skin wrinkles and the sag of flesh by toning up tissues. Special electrodes are available with which to target particular muscle groups and, by stimulating them selectively, you can go through a process of what actors and actresses call "facial gymnastics".

Remember, the SCENAR is capable of revitalizing the whole body and good energies always benefit the complexion!

It can even reduce scars or at least cause them to fade and become less visible.

One available attachment for the DENAS range is the DENS-glasses. T main device is connected to a set of goggles which contain metal stimulus probes. These deliver the bioresonance field right to the eyes and optic pathways and are said to benefit visual acuity, as well as ocular conditions.

THE THERAPEUTIC BLANKET

On a slightly separate issue you might notice that many sellers of SCENAR devices also offer a multilayer therapeutic healing blanket. These were invented by A.A.Datchenko of the Victoria company (http://www.odeialo.ru/) who also licensed other producers including OKB Ritm. They are approved by the Russian Ministry of Health and apparently very effective.

There are a number of pseudoscientific claims for this therapeutic adjunct. William Reich and his unsubstantiated orgone theory are often invoked. This I feel is nonsense and misleading. What seems clear to me is that the blankets:

- reflect the body's own far infrared healing radiations and so bathe the body in additional supportive energies
- reflects back biological extreme high frequency (EHF) radiations generated by the cells and organs in the range of 30 to 300 GHz
- Reflects away exogenous man-made EMF fields which might be harmful and which, as I indicated in chapter 10, have gradually become dangerous in intensity

All this relates far more closely to the work of Georges Lakhovsky and cellular radiations, visited in chapter 2, than it does to the tenuous theories of Reich. Remember, Lakhovsky taught that whichever radiation wins, that is what will happen to the tissues. So shielding the body from unwanted radiation while intensifying what is good and natural can only be nurturing and healthy.

FAME AND INFAMY

I'd like to conclude this chapter with what must be the most dramatic SCENAR case history ever told!

My friend Dr. Lorraine Ann Vanbergen-Haché was walking down a city street in the UK not long ago. Lori is an expert with the SCENAR. She was with a friend. It was down time. Suddenly a running man burst between them, followed closely behind by another, wielding an axe!

To the horror of the two women, right in front of them, the assailant buried the axe in the skull of the man he was chasing, threw away the weapon and ran off.

The victim collapsed to the ground, his skull cleaved open, revealing the meninges and brain. Yet, remarkably, he remained conscious.

Now Lori is a very calming individual and quickly took charge of the scene; asked someone to call an ambulance; demanded all the spectators be removed to a distance; and set to work. Her only tool was her SCENAR, which she carries in her purse at all times.

Lori worked around the wound, hoping to minimize the bleeding and damage, possibly also to sooth the energy field of a murder attack and the "information" imprint of violent damage to one of the body's most critical areas.

In due course the ambulance arrived. The paramedics could not believe the victim was even alive, never mind conscious, given the savage wound he had sustained. There had been almost no blood loss. The paramedics initiated standard procedure and whisked the wounded man off to the ER.

My friend Lori later visited the hospital to see the man she had saved and found him fully conscious. He was in some pain, not surprisingly, but filled with gratitude.

Just a story? Not at all: the entire event had been captured by a street surveillance video camera and everyone in the country was startled to see the tape replayed, showing the whole murderous attack and the strange woman who produced what looked like a TV remote from her purse and started rubbing it over the victim's head!

Lori was welcomed home that evening as a heroine, before she even realized that her quick-thinking action had been televised for all to see.[4]

Dr. McCoy ("Bones") would have been proud of her.

CHAPTER 12

WEIRD OR WHAT?

Right at the start of the 20th century, the biggest single risk factor for death due to heart disease was tooth and jaw infections. Numerous pathology specimens in medical school museums, showing sub-acute bacterial endocarditis, cavernous sinus thrombosis and brain abscesses, testify to just how precarious life could be in the age before antibiotics (and also what we may be facing again if we go on abusing them foolishly). A single unhealthy tooth could lead to an early grave. Now, at the very end of the century, what do you suppose is among the biggest predictors of death due to heart disease?

Teeth. Well, more exactly, gum disease. This one risk factor has recently been shown to be just as important as smoking, obesity, blood pressure or an unfortunate family history in determining whether you or I will die before we should.[1] This seems very new and startling. Yet it has been talked about by EAV practitioners for decades and by switched-on dentists like Weston Price for even longer than that. Why is what goes on in your mouth so dangerous?

Well, as my holistic dentist friend John Roberts, secretary of the British chapter of the International Academy of Oral Medicine and Toxicology, points out, teeth sockets are a royal highway for disease pathogens leading straight into your bones. If we were to piece together all the patches of infection that a dentist sees in a typical mouth, he tells me it would be the equivalent of an ulcer eating away at half the back of your hand. Would you stand for that? Of course not, you say. But that's exactly what most of us are doing – we just don't see it in our jaw bones.

A tooth abscess is really just another kind of osteomyelitis – that is, bacterial bone infection. We take the condition of our teeth far too lightly. No-one in his or her right mind would allow a hole to be drilled into a femur or other bone and have it left draining to the outside world; serious infectious complications would be bound to ensue. Yet that is what we do with our teeth; some people live with what is virtually an open wound.

The position is not helped by techniques such as the crowning of teeth. It may make them appear cosmetically attractive on the outside. But often these metal or plastic caps do nothing more than cover and hide a seat of purulent infection, waiting to explode at some time in the future when the body's defences are compromised.

In an address on 'The Role of Sepsis and Antisepsis in Medicine' to the Faculty of Medicine at McGill University, Montreal, in 1910, Dr William Hunter baited his colleagues by saying, 'Knowing as we do the pathogenic qualities of staphylococci and streptococci, we have not the slightest excuse for allowing the mouth, so easily accessible to local measures, to remain the chief seat and a veritable hotbed for their development and propagation; on the contrary, it is a severe reflection on our profession if we allow it.'[2]

Elsewhere, in a piece in the *Lancet*, the enlightened Hunter referred to gold fillings, gold caps, gold bridges, gold crowns and fixed dentures built in, on and around diseased teeth as 'a veritable *mausoleum* of gold'. I feel sure he chose the word advisedly.

BACK PRESSURE

The late Patrick Stortebecker, Professor of Neurology at the Karolinska Institute in Stockholm, Sweden, carried out a series of experiments in the 1960s which I consider highly illuminating. The results were also rather scary.

Stortebecker injected tooth bone margins under pressure with radio-opaque dyes and then took x-rays of the skull. What he showed was that most head veins do not have valve control and therefore blood could travel backwards into the cranium; his radio-opaque dye appeared all over the head, far away from the tooth in which was injected. Obviously this effect will take place in life; all it needs is for a change of pressure gradient, which is what happens every time you sneeze or strain at stool. This was a controlled hygienic experiment, but if the tooth in question should happen to be infected, the results could be very adverse indeed. Bacterial toxic matter could be propelled into the cranium and there set up an unwanted focus of infection right inside the skull.[3] Stortebecker himself mentioned the obvious risk of cavernous sinus thrombosis and suppuration. This was once a killer condition. The cavernous sinus is a large vein reservoir at the base of the brain, and if it should clot and become filled with purulent matter, widespread meningitis and brain abscesses were the almost inevitable result. Many fatal tragedies from nose picking and spot scratching took place in former times; those of us old enough may remember that parents tended to frown on this behaviour and we were slapped. Now you know there was a scientific reason for the almost universal injunction against spot scratching.

We no longer see this morbid condition in Western medicine, thankfully. But it lurks just beyond view, always a threat from dental infections, averted simply by the use of antibiotics. If we should lose the availability of an effective non-toxic antibiotic, as seems very probable the way they are being over-prescribed and pushed by drug companies, then worrying times will return.

But that's not all. Stortebecker had another disease model which I find very persuasive. He considers that what he found is the principal factor in the pathogenesis of multiple sclerosis.[4] Through extensive research he was able to show that most plaques of nerve de-myelination (the unmistakable sign of MS) were located around blood vessels. No-one else had noticed this important fact before. Stortebecker speculated that the back-pressure on veins had shunted toxic matter into the brain tissues, where it set up foci of inflammation and myelin loss. What was particularly convincing was that MS cases with optic neuritis (leading to blindness) generally had bad teeth and inflammation plaques in the brain; whereas those who had leg weakness or paralysis, with de-myelination plaques in the spinal cord, had pelvic or other lower-body disease foci. EAV folk find that the pelvic organs in particular hide a great deal of smouldering pathology. I myself have started to speak of a woman's 'angry pelvis', it is so common and so much undermines a woman's well-being.

Unfortunately, Stortebecker is gone. Apart from a handful of us, his work is ignored and it is very difficult to interest anyone in the medical establishment. Dentists don't even want to think about it. Doctors say it's a dental problem and nothing to do with them. Thus we have here another sad example of how specialization can make medicine ineffective. But the possibility that this hypothesis is sound requires that it be investigated scientifically, with adequate funding and proper protocol.

Just don't hold your breath.

TOXIC DENTISTRY

It is not really stretching the human mind too far to suggest that most dentistry is, by its nature, quite toxic. Modern methods rely heavily on materials such as metals, plastics and polymers, ceramics and prosthetic structures of many kinds. Unfortunately, EAV practitioners are discovering that most of this foreign material is stressful to the body. It can be a considerable drain on the immune system and therefore a major contributory cause of fatigue and chronic ill-health. In this new context we can only urge people even more emphatically to try to prevent dental problems from starting up. Good diet and adequate teeth hygiene may, even in this day of antibiotics, still be a key life-saver.

I do not exaggerate.

COOKED TEETH

Recent research by Ralph Turk and Fritz Kronner in Germany has shown that even the act of drilling a tooth causes severe energy disturbance.[5] Turk describes the modern dental turbine rotor as a sort of time-bomb, and that its damaging intensity has been completely missed by the vast majority of dentists. There are many likely reasons for this damage, not least being the fact that, despite water cooling, the temperature of the dentine rises by as much as 10 degrees after just a few *seconds* of drilling. In biological terms this is cooking the tooth. This denaturation obviously destroys the viability of the tooth and its ability to resist bacterial invasion. From over 6,000 cases studied it was uniformly seen that, as soon as a tooth was visited by a high-speed drill, focal osteitis trouble began in connection with that tooth within 2 years.

It is possible to reduce the damage by taking sensible anti-tox procedures before, during and after a dental programme. EAV tests show that this at least minimizes the impact of high-tech dentistry. Such elementary measures would include taking vitamin C, charcoal (to absorb toxins), homeopathic support and immune drainage remedies such as HEEL's lymphomyosot or Pascoe's Pascotox (Chapter 7 covers complex homeopathy).

MERCURY

Then there is the mercury story. Just over a decade ago, most of us were still to be convinced of the problem of biological intoxication with mercury. Official bodies such as the British and American Dental Associations deny it still.

As I said in my last book, gram for gram, mercury is one of the most toxic substances known to humanity, and it is arguably the most serious environmental pollutant we are creating for ourselves. Unfortunately mercury, especially in the methyl or chloride forms which have great biological penetration, has a special affinity for brain tissue. Most people know that the expression 'mad as a hatter' comes from the fact that twitching and dementia were once common among hat manufacturers and were due to poisoning with the mercuric nitrate used for curing felt hat bands.

The first health scare of modern times was the discovery that in the 1950s children who were dying of pink disease were being poisoned by mercury in 'teething powders'. Then, in 1953, the inhabitants of the Japanese fishing port of Minamata began to fall ill with a mysterious illness which caused twitching, mental confusion, difficulty in speaking and eventually paralysis. Autopsy showed considerable brain damage and the agent was discovered to be mercury. A nearby factory was dumping mercuric waste into the bay, which contaminated the fish stocks. It was concentrated in the food chain and reached deadly levels before being eaten by humans.

Despite all this, the dental profession continues to insist mercury is somehow non-toxic when you put it in your mouth! There is considerable hypocrisy about this, however; the instructions to dentists for handling mercury leave no doubt that it is harmful to dentists – even though it is supposed to be safe for patients. Advice to the profession includes storing it under water, not touching it by hand, providing adequate air extraction to eliminate the toxic vapour, and so on. Generally it is illegal for dentists to allow fluids contaminated by mercury to be sent into the sewage system. Filters or extractors are required.

The official argument was once that mercury remains firmly in the teeth and cannot spread to other tissues. Then in 1989 a team of doctors in Calgary, Canada, under Drs Hahn and Vimy, proved that the truth was very different. Using radioactive mercury and placing fillings in the teeth of sheep, they were able to show that mercury from fillings spreads all over a mammalian body *within hours*. The official line then switched to saying that there was no proven connection between mercury poisoning from amalgams and any known disease. This is specious and dishonest. It is not the public's job to prove there is a danger from mercury; it is the manufacturer's responsibility to show that it is safe. There is no prospect of this being possible.

The reason that the precipitating role of amalgams in disease processes is being missed is that doctors do not ask the right question: have you ever visited your primary care physician with a complaint and been asked 'Have you recently had any dental treatment?' Naturally, not. If doctors did check this important point they would be shocked at how often the answer would be yes.

What EAV doctors have been finding for years is that heavy metal overloads are a common cause of pathology and, not surprisingly, mercury is the godfather of all. Time and again mercury fillings are at the head of what I described in Chapter 8 as Causal Chains. However, this is not confined to mercury. Poisoning from other metals can occur. Sometimes the question is one of sensitivity, rather than poisoning.

We must accept what Nature tells us, and on testing a male patient with the Acupro I found that the biggest Indicator Drop pointed to danger from a gold-filled tooth and *not* the more obvious opposing amalgam. Scanning the dental nosode list showed that this patient was unusual in reacting to gold. I prescribed a homeopathic detoxification treatment and, next day, the gold filling fell out. Clearly it was rejected by the body, once given a little energetic help. The bemused patient preferred to believe it was 'just a coincidence', even though the tooth had remained in place for almost 20 years.

GALVANIC FIELDS AND ENERGETIC DISTURBANCE

Slightly more bizarre is the phenomenon of electrical fields around certain teeth and the effects these produce. I remember well the first time I saw Hal Huggin's slides of teeth cut open to show the scorch marks, where electrical current had been running for many years. Teeth can work like little batteries. This is quite logical: there are two or more metals and a saltwater fluid medium (saliva). This is how Allessandro Volta's original batteries were made; the battery of your motorcar is essentially the same thing.

The trouble starts from the fact that electrical currents actually leach the mercury out of the teeth, because of an effect called electrolysis. This is why patients sometimes complain of a constant metallic taste in the mouth, made worse by hot fluids and salty food (more electrolysis). If that isn't scary enough, then the reader should know that electrolysis is capable of releasing deadly mercury vapour. This goes straight to the brain tissue where it is highly invasive and toxic.

But the problem is even more complicated. The currents generated by amalgams can be quite considerable, and these are being formed very close to brain tissue, which operates at far lower potentials (a few millivolts). I have seen momentary spikes of up to 1 volt when testing teeth for the battery effect; this is enough to light a small torch battery. Remember the brain is really only a few millimetres from the jaw bone where the roots of the teeth lie, just the other side of the thin cranial bone and the meninges.

Thus there is potential for mental dysfunction and this is often found in clinical practice, if the appropriate questions are asked.

Casebook: Female, 44 Years

The patient had suffered from Meniere's disease: vertigo and vomiting, with intermittent staggering (sailor's gait). She could not think clearly any more, had trouble with her memory, could not see clearly – lines appeared not straight. This was accompanied by pain in the nape of the neck. She was unable to continue working, due to the severity of these symptoms. Her attending physicians could find no clinical explanation and the patient was told it was all in her head (in a way this was true!). Finally, a brain tumour was suspected and tests were required to exclude this grim possibility.

The patient's luck eventually turned and an ENT surgeon referred her to Dr Helmut Raue, an EAV specialist who understands biological dentistry, as this new speciality is called. He measured her teeth galvanically and found 215 microamperes of current between a gold filling and a nearby amalgam. One week after having the amalgam removed, all pain had disappeared and the patient's balance had returned to normal. The patient admitted then that she had had suicidal thoughts because of the excruciating pain and baffling dizziness.[6]

The reason that not enough of these cases are being diagnosed and the true picture not emerging is that patients do not, usually, consult their dentist with symptoms such as headache, facial neuralgia, dizziness, sleep disorders and digestive disturbance (just to give a few examples).

ENERGETIC FIELDS

EAV practitioners are finding teeth foci as a common cause of energetic disturbance. The problem is immensely more complicated than it at first might seem. Several key acupuncture meridians cross the line of the teeth as they pass over the face. An abscess or 'transmitting focus' can actually create pathological results anywhere along the line of that meridian. These are further connected with secondary organs and sites. Thus problems with a front incisor tooth may impact on the kidneys, since this meridian passes through the incisors. But the kidneys, in turn, are related to the knee joints. If I see a patient with incisor problems or a bridge in this location I can surprise him or her by asking about the arthritis of the knees.

Sometimes the consequences of these interconnections are very surprising and virtually beggar explanation but should make us very wary indeed about the effects of dentistry.

Casebook: Female, 33 Years

A dentist had prepared a new crown tooth prosthesis, the type with a post of nickel which fits in a hole drilled down the centre of the tooth to give support. As the dentist offered the post to its new location on the right upper jaw, the woman let out a squeal: she'd gone immediately blind in that eye! The dentist removed the tooth and she could see again. He offered it back and she went blind again. This was repeated several times until both were quite sure of what they were observing.

She refused the crown and had the tooth removed instead.

What this striking case example of what we might call 'virtual dentistry' tells us is that energetic fields in the mouth are important to brain function. This was an *instant* reaction; there was no way it could depend on any chemical manifestation, even metal toxicity. Allergies to nickel do occur, though this metal is far less poisonous than mercury. But any such allergy would take a little time to develop. The striking part of the story is the *instant* loss of vision, which indicates clearly neurological dysfunction along the optical pathways due to a field disturbance, probably at the quantum or information level.

It also makes vividly clear what risks we take when we allow metal into our mouths. The resulting disturbance of the body's energy field can have unpredictable and very seri-

ous consequences. *I try to imagine in this case what would
have happened if the woman had not lost her vision immediately but had gone blind over the subsequent few weeks.*
Almost certainly the correct cause would never have been
diagnosed. She may have ended up with harmful and unnecessary interventions which would fail because they were
not aimed at correcting the real problem.

ENERGETIC MERIDIAN RELATIONS WITH TEETH

Figure 11 shows the main teeth relations with acupuncture
meridians revealed by EAV. There are charts published which
give a great deal of detail about these biological dental inter-rela-
tionships, but I have tried to simplify this down to the general
picture for the reader.

ENERGETIC RELATIONSHIPS OF TEETH

	upper	relations
1	incisor	kidney, bladder, pineal, rectum
2	incisor	kidney, bladder, pineal, rectum
3	canine	liver, gallbladder, pituitary, posterior eye
4	pre-molar	lung, colon, posterior pituitary
5	pre-molar	lung, colon, thymus
6	1st molar	spleen/pancreas, stomach, thyroid
7	2nd molar	spleen/pancreas, stomach, parathyroid
8	3rd molar	heart, small intestine, anterior pituitary
	lower	**relations**
4	pre-molar	spleen/pancreas, stomach, gonads
5	pre-molar	spleen/pancreas, stomach, breast
6	1st molar	lung, colon
7	2nd molar	lung, colon
8	3rd molar	heart, small intestine, ext/middle ear

note how upper and lower jaw reverse relations on teeth 4- 7

NICO: WHAT'S IN A NAME?

NICO is an EAV disease. By that I mean only EAV people would usually detect this curious type of pathology. It's a dental problem and has only come to light recently as a result of dentists doing their own EAV testing, though in fairness other good dentists do come across it.

NICO is an abbreviation of neuralgia-inducing cavitational osteonecrosis. I will explain. First, let me remind you that disease under the roots of teeth is a kind of bone inflammation, hence the term 'osteitis'. Osteonecrosis means the bone has died or lost its viability as a result; it is softened and eaten away, like rot in an apple. Neuralgia-inducing means that it has been postulated as a potent cause of neuralgia of the face, particularly that vicious kind known as trigeminal neuralgia. The trigeminal nerve (5th cranial nerve, emerging at the ear) is largely sensory and supplies the face, jaws and teeth. A phenomenon known as referred pain means that trouble anywhere within the nerve net can be felt at other places supplied by the same nerves. Thus NICO is a factor to consider in migraine or any kind of atypical headache. It is worth pointing out that the jaws are the only major bony tissue with important sensory nerve endings.

The 'cavitational' part of the name simply means some kind of cyst or space in the jaw bone, not necessary infected or inflammatory. Quite common is a fatty osteitis, where an old focus of inflammation has finally settled down and turned into a fatty cyst. There may be blood or chocolate matter in the cavity. But the important point which knowledgeable dentists are making is that this is not really an inflammatory process but tissue destruction caused by insidious loss of blood supply. In this respect it is more like other textbook bone diseases, where destruction comes from impaired blood and nutritional supply, which in 1915 US dentist G. V. Black described as progressive 'death of bone, cell by cell'.[7]

NICO is not rare. In one population study it was found in 1 in every 4,900 adults. This makes NICO by far the most common osteonecrotic bone disease; once again, specialization means that doctors are not talking to dentists as they should. NICO has been seen in people aged 18–94, but typically affects people in the 35–65 age range. An individual may have more than one focus of this disease process. It is hard to avoid the conclusion that it is the result of poor dental hygiene and maintenance; in other words, the consequence of burnt-out chronic infective foci.

Whatever the primary cause, bone cavities are open to subsequent bacterial invasions. Because the underlying process is caused by lack of oxygen these are likely to be anaerobic bacteria which release dangerous toxins and may in our present view be pre-malignant. Substances such as mercaptan and thioether, which are found regularly in dental foci by electro-dermal screening (EDS), are known carcinogens. It is unfortunate that NICO is usually not visible on x-ray. Many cases are missed even by experienced diagnosticians, since 35–50 per cent of bone loss is necessary before changes become radiographically evident. This is where EAV and virtual dentistry come in. I know dentists who are bold enough, and trust good EAV practitioners sufficiently, to drill into bone at the site indicated as a reading focus. It is very satisfying to both parties when the cortex is breached and a cavity filled with biological sludge makes its presence known.

Once diagnosed, treatment is currently by curettage of the site, sweeping away all the dead and softened bone, and maybe the first millimetre or so of healthy bone, in the hope that new, good bone will form. Coral granules may be used to pack the hole and encourage re-calcification of bone tissue. In about a third of cases this radical treatment fails and may even make the problem worse, but according to one writer only about 10 per cent of patients feel that the process wasn't worthwhile. Curettage is rather heroic and I have no doubt that in future something a little less aggressive will be the rule. While NICO is chiefly the domain of holistic dentists, such 'commando cures' are rather untypical of holism in general.

ROOT CANAL FILLINGS

Here is a topic where conventional medicine, decades ago, stood right where alternative innovative dentists stand today. The story is a fascinating one and begins in the first decade of this century with one Dr Billings. His research, published in 1914, showed that 95 per cent of all focal infections in the body came from the teeth and tonsils. Billing's work, in turn, was found by Weston Price, a leading dentist of his day. Price was an advocate of a healthy natural lifestyle and keynote nutrition; in every way he was a great thinker and a pioneer of values that we cherish today.

Price had a woman patient for whom he had done a root canal filling. She subsequently developed bad arthritis; it was so severe that she had become bedridden most of the time and her hands were so badly swollen she could barely feed herself. Price was honest enough to ask the question that no dentist cares to ask: could he have made her ill systemically by propagating generalized infection, as Billings had shown? He removed the root-canal-filled tooth, carefully and aseptically, to see what would happen. The woman promptly recovered.

From this case forward Price became very interested in the problem of root canal fillings. He had considerable success in helping patients, and published his results widely. There are copious papers by him in the medical and dental literature, most of it from the early 1920s. It is important to recognize that Price was a leading conventional dentist of the day. His views were listened to and, for a time, it became the fashion among doctors to recommend extracting teeth with root canal fillings as a cure for arthritis.

In fact this progressed to widespread tooth extractions, root canals or not, which was not what Price originally taught. Unfortunately, many cases did not recover as expected. The patient not only continued to suffer the arthritis but was now without any teeth. The approach became unpopular and was eventually discontinued. As a result, Price's views were discredited and lost sight of. It was one of those cases where the pendulum swung too far in a particular direction. Price was right, of course, but there needed to be some way of choosing patients who would benefit from removing root canal fillings.

Voll gave us the means. It is now a common aspect of EDS diagnosis to consider the safety and validity of root canal fillings. They may not be a problem. If the person is fit and strong, with a good immune system, the situation can continue unchanged for many years. But if at some time in the future he or she undergoes too much stress or suffers from a major illness, resistance may be compromised and the dangers of root canals become manifest and dangerous.

The problem is that, although root canal work looks fine on x-ray and it might appear that there is a perfect occlusion of the former root canal down the heart of the tooth, microscopic examination reveals a different story. Tooth dentine, which is hard and screeches like rock when the dentist attacks it with his drill, is really composed of numerous tiny tubules. It is said there are 3 miles of end-to-end tubules in every tooth; they are supposed to conduct nutrients to keep the tooth alive and healthy. When bacteria gain access to the tooth, they lurk in these tubules. Filling the root canal does not flush the pathogens out of this domain. In fact the bacteria are then trapped in a closed-off space and inevitably cause trouble.

Pathogens have to go somewhere when they multiply. They can migrate through what are called lateral tubules and escape into the periodontal membrane and subsequently into the bony tissue of the jaw. From there they migrate around the body. As biological dentist and author of *Root Canal Cover Up*[8] George Meinig puts it:

> These bacteria are kind of like people, if they get to like Seattle or Reno or someplace they decide that's where they are going to have their home. Well, the bacteria travelling round the body, they may get to the liver, the kidneys or the heart or eyes or some other tissue and they set up an infection in that area. This is why the degenerative diseases occur from the teeth.[9]

TRANSMITTING TEETH

Now we come to the part that is definitely weird, hence the title of this chapter. Everything so far is at least logical, if rather unnerving. It makes sense. From here it makes no real sense, except in the insubstantial quantum domain or, as we would once have said, 'the etheric'. What Weston Price did in the 1920s was to take infected and pathogenic root-canal-filled teeth and surgically stitch them into rabbits for observation. This is an example of one of those experimental situations like Benjamin Franklin sending his kite up into a thunderstorm: a mixture of perverse genius and intuition that leads to some important scientific insight.

What Weston Price found was that the rabbits became ill with the same diseases as the patients, or if not exactly the same diseases, then the same organ was attacked in some way. If the human had nephritis (cured after tooth extraction), then the rabbit got nephritis; if the human had heart disease, cancer or arthritis, that was what the rabbit got. Eye problems were particularly striking; if the human had only mild eye trouble, the rabbit would react so severely as to go blind in two or three days.

The only real conclusion is that the tooth carried some message of disease using an unknown code. Whether it was a quantum field factor or some other means of information transference is simply not known. You would think this absolutely fascinating series of experiments would have scientists racing to investigate the significance of what Price found. Instead, his work was promptly forgotten for over 50 years. So much for the progress of scientific thought.

WHAT YOU CAN DO

You might be worried about what is written here. This could be with good cause, but don't over-react. The first thing to do is make contact with a biological dentist, as they call themselves. These are advanced dentists who appreciate Price's work and freely use homeopathic remedies, nutrition and other natural accompaniments to dental hygiene. They also willingly interact with EAV practitioners, preferring the body's own signals for guidance.

Read more and become informed about the issues. Everyone should take responsibility for their own health care and this applies equally to dentistry. To leave decisions solely to your dentist, if he or she is of conventional thought mode, is to be subject to yesterday's science and it may do you harm in the long run, as we have seen with the mercury story (there remain dentists who *still* insist there is no problem with mercury amalgams).

Eat a proper diet which avoids sugars that cause dental decay and feed micro-organisms. Increase your intake of alkalizing foods to counter any chronic acidosis problem, as discussed in Chapter 11.

Use co-enzyme Q10 supplements (ubiquinone). This has been shown to have unequivocal benefit for periodontal (gum) disease. More teeth are lost due to gum disease than decay (cavities).

Large doses of vitamin C seem to be very helpful for periodontal disease and toxicity of all kinds. Take large amounts before, during and after any dental programme – at least 10 g (2½ teaspoonsful) daily.

CHAPTER 13

THE NON-MATERIAL
NATURE OF SUBSTANCES

In keeping with the spirit of this book I began a lecture tour in 2001 (which I still give) entitled: "The Non-Material Nature of Substances and Medicines".

In it I take a major accepted hypothesis and show it to be false: *Only weighable substances with a rest mass and a sufficient biochemical gradient can affect biological organisms.* In other words there has to be substances present and in sufficient quantity, for there to be any measurable biological effect. All of medical science is based on this idea, which is assumed to be a "given".

It is not.

The truth, which I prove three times over, using different modalities, is that unweighable (nonmaterial) substances have profound measurable biological effects and that this may even be the paramount mechanism. If that is correct then it must also apply to medicines and remedies.

It must also shake so-called "scientific medicine" to its very foundations!

You have the first argument on page 14, in which I cited a study which showed that lithium did not need to be present, if the lithium conditions of cyclotron resonance were met. Rats were sedated by the electromagnetic signal, even though no actual substance (no rest mass) was actually present. Yet cyclotron resonance is a phenomenon of classical physics. Its quantum counterpart, nuclear magnetic resonance, has all the additional mysteries of non-locality etc. Neither of these 100% scientific phenomena require any actual substance: just the unique energetic signal.

If the audience is a little stiff on this revelation, I like to point out that although it was first "discovered" nearly a century ago by Albert Abrams, that same cyclotron resonance effect has now reached conventional medicine. Did you know that the famous Mayo clinic has installed a cyclotron resonance detector? It's really the same as Abram's "black box" detector—just more sophisticated, much more expensive and blessed with the credibility of up-to-date science. They call it a Fourier Transform Ion Cyclotron Resonance Mass Spectrometer or "FT-ICR mass spec" for short.

So I am pleased to boast that even in the few years since the first edition of this book, that the Mayo Clinic too has adopted "virtual medicine" as a modality.

Incidentally, nuclear magnetic resonance (NMR), which is a similar phenomenon but in the quantum domain, has been shown to apply at the macro- or biological level[1]. This is a significant breakthrough and overturns the traditional dogma that quantum events do not affect biological systems. NMR is capable of causing cataracts in the eye lens of cows and ox. It has also been shown that NMR can alter nutritional function, by interfering with the uptake and utilization of nutrient ions, exactly as I predicted in the first edition of Virtual Medicine. What's more a "memory of water" effect was shown, meaning the adverse effect could be migrated to other organisms and would begin to affect those too[2].

SERIAL DILUTIONS

The second case I use is homeopathy, which I introduced in chapter 7. One of the big problems that conventional scientists and doctors have with homeopathy is that most of the active therapeutic solutions are so dilute there is none of the original substances left. Once past the so-called "Avogadro number" or "Loschmidt number", which is a 1023 dilutions or 23 zeros, we know from simple chemistry that no molecules remain, since there are 1023 molecules in a standardized (molar) solution.

That sounds a lot but when homeopaths dilute 100 x100 x100 x100... they only have to do this 12 times (12C which is 12 followed by 24 zeros) and they have gone beyond the Avogradro number. 12C is actually not very dilute in homeopathic terms: solutions of 200C are used routinely or even 1000C (1M as it's called).

Nobody, not even me or the homeopaths, argue that some actual substance must remain present—there is none, truly. But that does not mean there can be no effect. We think of the substance's unique property as an energetic signal or, in the very high dilutions, pure information. This energy or information is "printed" on the water and so can be used therapeutically, long after the actual substance is gone.

Yet it isn't quite that simple; a poison will not remain a poison!

Notice that in the process of ultra-dilution, a toxic substance is transformed to being one of beneficial healing. Consider the homeopathic master remedy Lachesis, derived from the South American bushmaster snake, which is very venomous indeed. The symptoms of being bitten include a weak heart; a rapid, weak, irregular pulse; palpitations; angina; and difficulty in breathing— leading eventually to circulatory collapse and death. Yet these symptoms are the very ones eased by taking the very diluted form of the venom (Lachesis). This is rather wondrous to behold.

If you will recall the Arndt-Schulz Law I introduced on page 119, I explained that small doses of a substance can be beneficial but that larger doses act as a poison and shut down the system.

Turned around this means that even poisonous substances can be beneficial, if used in small enough quantities. Indeed strychnine, a deadly poison, was once used in bottled "tonics" which older readers will remember in the medicine cupboard. Instead of killing you it re-vitalized (ie. put life back in) you.

Now there is substantial proof from a different direction that, like it or not, homeopathically potentizing (diluting) a substance, even beyond the point where there is any physical molecules present, still creates a biochemical effect.

First, there were the South Korean chemists who discovered that molecules dissolved in water clump together as they get more diluted[3]. Furthermore, the size of the clumps depends on the history of dilution, making a mockery of the 'laws of chemistry'.

Then in 2003 Swiss physicist Louis Rey published the results of a startling experiment in Physica A, a reputable journal specialising in statistical mechanics. Rey was investigating the effect of sodium and lithium chloride on the dissociation of water molecules, using a well-established conventional technique called thermoluminescence.

In fact Rey used "heavy water" or deuterium hydroxide, since it performs better. When heated from deep frozen (77^0 Kelvin), irradiated deuterium gives off two distinct luminescence peaks: one around 122^0 K and the other at 166^0 K. Adding sodium chloride or lithium chloride enhances this process and results in a larger dissociation.

That's all very mainstream. But in a fit of curiosity (which could have cost him his job!) Rey decided to see what happened if he used only homeopathically diluted sodium or lithium chloride. He followed the proper procedure, including succession (shaking) between dilutions, and went to a dilution way beyond the Avogadro number, which the reader will now be aware means that no physical substance remains.

The results? Exactly the same! Homeopathically prepared substances, diluted beyond the presence of any weighable rest mass, still created a potent physico-chemical effect[4]. Predictably, Rey has been attacked and criticized, just as Benveniste was.

Martin Chaplin from London's South Bank University, an expert on water and hydrogen bonding, for instance, claims "Rey's rationale for water memory seems most unlikely." Chaplin suggests that tiny amounts of impurities in the samples, perhaps due to inefficient mixing, could be getting concentrated at the boundaries between different phases in the ice and causing the changes in thermoluminescence. This is mere speculative comment, of course, disguised as science.

Contrast Chaplin's shaky intellectual position with that of thermoluminescence expert Raphael Visocekas from the Denis Diderot University of Paris. Visocekas took the trouble to visit Rey and watched him carry out some of his experiments.

"The experiments showed a very nice reproducibility," Visoce-kas told New Scientist. "It is trustworthy physics."[5]

Just be patient. In time, as with Benveniste's memory of water, the results will be repeated and confirmed quietly in many independent universities.

But the critics of homeopathy, like Prof. Edzard Ernst, will ignore these later findings and go on spouting their dogma that "there is no proof" that homeopathy works.

THE DIGITIZED "SIGNATURE" OF MATERIAL SUBSTANCES

The third proof of my Virtual Medicine hypothesis lies also in the work of the late Jacques Benveniste, which you can review in chapter 7.

It rests with the fact that when atoms come together they form a molecule held together energy bonds which both emit and absorb certain specific electromagnetic frequencies. No two species of molecule have the same electromagnetic oscillations or energetic signature.

Benveniste was able to show that these characteristics of a biochemical substance did not depend on its physical presence but could be replicated digitally and used to "inform" water. This informed water would then generate the characteristic response attributable to the substance in question: but there was no trace of the physical substance present in the test medium.

The technicalities are challenging but need not concern the average reader. Basically, the substance under review was turned into a digital (binary) signal, using a transducer via an ordinary computer sound card (I think he told me, or I read, he used an ordinary Soundblaster card).

Once in the form of an electronic file, the "substance signature" or EMS as he called it (electromagnetic signal) could be handled like any other computer file. It could be burned to a floppy disc, attached to an e-mail or sent via the Internet as a download.

A typical experiment of this type would proceed as follows:

A quantity of the substrate would be obtained, say phorbol myristate acetate (PMA), a useful test agent capable of generating reactive oxygen metabolites (ROM) or "free radicals". This was then turned into an electromagnetic signature file.

Using a transducer, water would be treated or "informed" with the PMA file, played to it through a transducer. This could be compared to the effect (if any) of plain water as a control. The effect of real PMA was known and, as a further investigation, the team tested whether SOD (superoxidase dismutase), a substance known to block reactive oxygen species, had any detectable effect.

Results were tested by measuring production of reactive oxygen metabolites (ROM). The reader will be pleased to hear these studies were very reproducible and measurements of ROM consistently showed identical effects, whether the chemical substances used was "real" or digitized water.[6]

It is very satisfying that the SOD blocked ROM release, even by the "informed" or digitized water. This suggests to me at least the probability that the real mechanism of most biochemical reactions is that of electromagnetic signaling and not "stuff" interacting with other "stuff" at all!

Later as well as replicating these results elsewhere Benveniste and colleagues at the Northwestern University in Chicago were able to send digitized biological information via telephone, on a floppy disc, via the Internet, even as an e-mail attachment and still replicate the effects at the other end .[7]

THE BIRTH OF DIGITAL BIOLOGY

Benveniste has successfully given birth to a whole new paradigm he christened "digital biology". It's going to be a rough ride getting it accepted in the die-hard community of people who believe utterly in the untenable model of biochemical collisions as the basis for life (that's how molecules are supposed to signal to each other).

Follow along with Benveniste in his own words:

Life depends on signals exchanged among molecules. For example, when you get angry, adrenalin "tells" its receptor, and it alone (as a faithful molecule, it talks to no other) to make your heart beat faster, to contract superficial blood vessels, etc..

In biology, the words "molecular signal" are used very often. Yet, if you ask even the most eminent biologists what the physical nature of this signal is, they seem not even to understand the question, and stare at you wide-eyed. In fact, they've cooked up a rigorously Cartesian physics all their own, as far removed as possible from the realities of contemporary physics, according to which simple contact (Descarte's laws of impact, quickly disproved by Huygens) between two coalescent structures creates energy, thus constituting an exchange of information.

For many years, I believed and recited this catechism without realizing its absurdity, just as mankind did not realize the absurdity of the belief that the sun circles the earth.

The truth, based on facts, is very simple. It does not require any "collapse of the physical or chemical worlds." That molecules vibrate, we have known for decades. Every atom of every molecule and every intermolecular bond-the bridge that links the atoms-emits a group of specific frequencies. Specific frequencies of simple or complex molecules are detected at distances of billions of light-years, thanks to radio-telescopes. Biophysicists describe these frequencies as an essential physical characteristic of matter, but biologists do not consider that electromagnetic waves can play a role in molecular functions themselves. We cannot find the words "frequency" or "signal" (in the physical sense of the term) in any treatise on molecular interactions in biology.

[from his website www.digibio.com "Understanding Digital Biology; accessed 4/15/2008 at 2.18 PDT]

Doesn't this echo the words of Georges Lahkovsky, chapter 2, p 20, "'I have been attacked by physicists ignorant of biology and by biologists ignorant of physics who consequently can neither understand my theories nor judge my experiments'?

I too was raised on the old-fashioned view of "lock and key" molecular activity and believed in it utterly at the time. So I know how deeply entrenched this model has become. That's the problem. It's like wearing glasses: you don't see the lenses, just the view beyond (altered by the different focus).

But, like Benvensite, I'm as sure today it's wrong I was sure then it was correct.

Let's compare the two models and see which is more plausible. First, the background to the digital biology model:

- All cells communicate via molecular resonance
- mutual resonance extends outwards, like chain reactions, spreading to other molecules nearby (just like piano strings vibrate when something nearby excites them!)
- All fields extend to the ends of the universe, even though they get fainter and fainter (basic physics)
- Almost instant (speed of light)
- every substance known to have characteristic frequencies which, theoretically, can be detected right across the universe

The traditional model, on the other hand, relies on molecules actually bumping into each other. I blush when I think I once believed this! It's almost impossible!

The more of a substance is present, the more likely a collision, that much I can agree with. This model has a technical name QSAR (quantitative structure activity relationship). In simpler terms we would say that it relies on a concentration gradient.

The QSAR model therefore has the following characteristics:

- needs direct contact
- relies on random collision
- uncontrolled, trial-and-error basis
- statistically virtually impossible
- the simplest biological event would require a very long time

The way I illustrate this in my public lectures is as follows:

Let's suppose we take 10,000 super elastic white tennis balls, which bounce almost indefinitely, and set them all in motion in the Carnegie Hall auditorium. Then we follow up by launching

100 yellow super elastic tennis balls, which are also in motion nearly indefinitely. How long do you think it would take before 2 of the yellow balls actually collided?

Well, the answer is that it could happen in the first 2 seconds. But it could also take a week. All we can say is, with precise probability math, we can predict the likely length of time it would take. I don't need to do that here; it's a very long time. Just follow the reasoning.

This reliance on chance encounter is virtually impossible for biological functioning. On a reasonable timescale, even for molecular-size systems, it's going to take too long. Or it would require a HUGE presence of the active substrate (a lot of the yellow balls). Yet we find in typical biological systems that concentrations of very active substrates (like hormones) are almost infinitesimally small, the equivalent of say 6 - 8 yellow balls among the 10,000 white ones.

Nevertheless there is an effect.

The digital model explains this easily:

Substances do not need to make contact, ever. The resonating field extends outwards to infinity (OK, classical physics resonance is going to peter out slowly with distance. But NMR is a quantum effect and therefore non-local).

Digital biology:
- requires no direct contact
- therefore distance not a problem
- resonance enabled by geomagnetic field
- instantaneous, which is often seen in medical biology.
- Extremely low frequencies work at very attenuated levels
- even high-frequency molecules can "beat" at an ELF

Let me explain the last two points, which to me are the clinchers.

The cyclotron resonance effect we began with in chapter 1 relies on a simple mathematical equation as follows: $\nu = (1/2\pi)(\rho/\varphi)\beta$. It probably looks scary but it isn't really. All the funny Geek letters in brackets are just math symbols, which can be substituted, giving the cyclotron resonance characteristics of any known substance. Just ignore them.

We only need to look at the $v = \beta$ elements of the equation. Those are saying that v (frequency) is directly proportional to β (the intensity). Turn that around and it means the lower the frequency, the lower the corresponding intensity needed to create an effect.

This is why extreme low frequencies are so powerful, biologically speaking. They need only a very low strength field to work! [relax, this ends the math!]

So you see even if the field was weak (not many yellow balls, or too far apart), it doesn't matter on this model. The molecules can still talk to each other.

Neat, isn't it?

Now the only bit we have left to clarify, in order for you to know 1,000 times more physics than your medical practitioner, is what I mean by "beats" and how that phenomenon fits into the picture.

Many molecules have quite high frequencies. They don't qualify as ELF. But simultaneous high frequencies which are close, but not identical, resonate with a very slow secondary rhythm which is the difference between the two frequencies. Stay with me for a moment: if you sounded a tuning fork at 440 cycles per second (middle "A") and then started off a second tuning fork doing only 443 cycles per second, you would hear a wu-wu-wu-wu-wu-wu "beat" of 3 cycles per second (perhaps you wouldn't hear it at first but with practice...).

In fact that's how orchestral musicians all tune their instruments together. They listen for beats and tune until the beats get slower and slower (less difference) and then finally the beats disappear altogether, meaning the two instruments are perfectly in tune.

In fact this is where the sound element comes in. Benveniste, you'll remember me saying was recording electromagnetic signatures via a computer sound card; well, now you know why. Many specific frequencies he was working with fall within the range of "sound" or the infrared spectrum.

DIAGNOSIS

But wait a minute! Could this signature idea be used to detect the presence of pathogenic substances and organisms? Maybe we could do away with the need for blood samples, biopsies and other physical sampling in order to make an accurate diagnosis?

You bet.

And in the course of time that may become Benveniste's greatest legacy.

In his Portakabin laboratory in Paris (all that was left to him after the "memory of water" debacle), he and his DigiBio team went on breaking the frontiers of science and medicine.

One of the headline studies involved a detection method for the bacteria E Coli, an occasional human pathogen. The K1 strain, particularly, is a major cause of enteric/diarrheal diseases, urinary tract infections, and sepsis.

In line with their previous work, the team electronically captured, digitized, and transmitted the specific electromagnetic signal (EMS) of the K1 bacteria to a biological system sensitive to that exact pathogen (or its EMS).

First they digitally recorded the EMS from E. Coli K1 and two other substances as controls: staphylococcus (3.5 million/ml) or saline.

Next, they set up latex particles, sensitized by a K1 antibody, from Pasteur Diagnostics. These particles will clump or aggregate in the presence of real E. Coli K1.

When the Staph EMS was played, little happened; when the control (saline) EMS was applied, little happened.

But the E. Coli K1 EMS induced the formation of significant aggregates (larger than that of Staphylococcus or saline).

What was curious – and here's the integrity of the man – is that Benveniste reported that the magnitude of aggregation varied from day to day. It was not consistent. Yet, always in comparison for the controls of that day, the team seldom made a mistake in separating E. Coli. This was repeated over hundreds of experiments[8].

This is remarkable in that a diagnostic test was performed with *none* of the pathogenic substance present, only it's electromagnetic "signature". Incidentally, these were common or garden ".wav" files, familiar to any computer literate individual.

As Benveniste remarks, since these signal files can travel a long distance, it should become possible to detect any immunogenic substance from a remote location.

Don't send blood or urine: send a .wav file!

So finally we are tying together all the strands from Albert Abram's reflexophone and oscilloclast, via the dermatron and Voll's EAV machines, to modern day computer analysis and digitized "specimens".

DIGITAL TREATMENT!

Remember, part of Abram's original discovery was that pathogens could be eliminated by playing them hostile frequencies, though his "Oscilloclast" (p. 8). What is the current state of play on this?

In chapter 6 I referred to so-called bioresonance therapy, where specific chosen frequencies can be played to the tissues, producing a therapeutic response. MORA machines, the BICOM and similar devices have now reached a state of sophistication where they are practically, in themselves, a new healing paradigm. Even the mighty little SCENAR (chapter 11) can be considered to belong to this family of healing devices.

But this would be a good place to introduce another electronic healing model, which is scandalously controversial (I love it), and at the same time fascinating and instructive in its scientific, biological and medical impact.

I'm referring to the work of Royal Raymond Rife.

It's an involved, bitterly disputed story, generally distorted with fanciful embroideries and has reached near mythic proportions in some accounts of his life and work. Moreover much of the supposed teaching and documentary material in circulation about Rife comes from people who are trying to promote their own me-too versions of the Rife machine and their documentary evidence is often suspect, to say the least.

Let's stick with the main therapeutic facts.

Rife was unarguably a brilliant technician. He was hired by Henry Timken, an industrial magnate, and under Timken's sponsorship produced the most technologically advanced speedboat marine engine of the day (1915), generating 2700 HP.

Rife went on with Timken's support to develop microscopes and almost perfected the art, producing compounded quartz prisms in a glycerine bath, which gave resolutions of up to 50,000 diameters; this was at a time when the best commercial laboratory microscopes could give only up to 2,000 diameters. Rife's Universal Microscope was without doubt the greatest optical instrument ever designed; no-one can seriously question this aspect of Rife's work.

It's what he SAW that started the acrimony and disputation.

BUT FIRST, HOW DID HE DO IT?

What was different about Rife's microscopes was not just the optics but the technique used to visualize living specimens, without killing them.

More than 75% of the organisms Rife could see with his Universal Microscope are only visible with ultra-violet light. Hence the quartz lenses and prisms: only quartz is transparent to UV light. But ultraviolet light is outside the range of human vision. Rife overcame this limitation by heterodyning, a technique which became popular in early radio broadcasting. Heterodyning is a fancy name for something we've already met, the way that two different frequencies will transfer their energy to a third "beat" frequency (now you know why I asked you to be patient and try to follow the complex, but necessary explanation).

Rife illuminated the microorganism (usually a virus or bacteria) with two different wavelengths of the same ultraviolet light frequency which resonated with the spectral signature of the microbe. These two wavelengths produced interference where they merged. This interference was, in effect, a third, longer wave which fell into the visible portion of the electromagnetic spectrum. This is exactly the same process by which Benveniste got his frequencies down to the human auditory range.

Rife painstakingly identified the individual spectroscopic signature of each microbe, using a slit spectroscope attachment. Then, he slowly rotated the block of quartz prisms to focus light of a single wavelength upon the microorganism he was examining (you will remember from high school physics that a prism splits white light into its component frequencies). The selected wavelength was chosen because it resonated with the spectroscopic signature frequency of the microbe based on the now-established fact that every molecule oscillates at its own distinct frequency (this was 50 - 60 years before Benveniste came across the same realization).

The result of using a resonant wavelength is that micro-organisms which are invisible in white light suddenly become visible in a brilliant flash of light when they are exposed to the color frequency that resonates with their own distinct spectroscopic signature, coordinating with the chemical composition of the organism. Rife likened this effect to using light as the equivalent of a chemical stain in conventional microbiology. In fact the particles Rife was able to visualize were smaller than the molecules of typical acid and aniline dye conventional stains!

This new technique gave Rife a unique advantage and enabled him to see things nobody had ever seen before with ordinary microscopes.

Rife became the first human being to actually scc a live virus, and until quite recently, his microscope was the only one which was able to view live viruses. Even more amazingly, he saw that when a Tubercle bacillus was destroyed, it split into many smaller living particles, he called TB viruses (a virus at that time was just considered to be a filterable bacterium).

These altered forms we call pleomorphism and it is bitterly disputed, even today, that such a thing can take place. Of course none of the experts who deny its existence has ever looked through a Rife microscope!

But Rife also saw something else, something startling, something that shouldn't be there!

THE NON-MATERIAL NATURE OF SUBSTANCES

BACILLUS X

Rife saw curious tiny little living virus-size organisms in the blood of cancer patients. They were too small to be bacteria but were not viruses. He found they gave off a distinctive purple-red emanation when viewed in the microscope. He named this entity bacillus X, or "BX" and claimed to have verified its existence in every instance of carcinoma he examined.

At that time virus causation of cancer was unheard of. Moreover it was not known that viruses were simply protein capsules containing either RNA or DNA. On our present model, BX was cancer trouble just waiting to happen. In fact Rife was able to convert from cancer to the organelle and back 104 times. He injected rats with the organelles and created cancers. These were then used to obtain more organelles and pass the disease on to the next rat and so. He did this 411 times in total, with the same result. Cancer was transferred by a small filterable moety he called "BX". That's pretty convincing.

He also found another organisms associated with sarcoma he called "BY".

But few were prepared to believe Rife. Despite widespread media of the day claiming that "The cure for cancer has been found", the idea of a cancer virus or cancer bacterium was too far beyond the boundaries of knowledge at the time (1932).

As well as general skepticism there was the orchestrated attack from lackeys of the Rockefeller family. Bitter wrangling and controversy broke out. It was obvious that vested interest and big dollars did not care about human health but merely in eliminating the threat to the medical monopoly posed by this new breakthrough.

LETHAL RAYS

Rife discovered that if you play a resonant frequency to an organism it will oscillate or vibrate with it, until it bursts, like the singer's trick of singing the specific note of a drinking glass and make it shatter. The same thing happened with cancer cells and other NO-NOs. This killing disruption was called electroporation, and led to the cell's immediate malfunction and death. The fatal frequency Rife termed the MOR or mortal oscillatory rate.

Now, here is another loop closed by this present text: Rife's early investigations were contemporaneous with that of the still-living Albert Abrams. Rife, it is known, actually had one of Abrams' Oscilloclasts (p. 8). From this prototype, Rife also designed and had constructed his own oscillator which was capable of generating a wider spectrum of individual frequencies than the Abrams' machine. By a painstaking process of examining the BX in culture while stepping through a wide array of frequencies, Rife found the one which "devitalized" it.

Rife isolated the organisms and found an MOR for tuberculosis, E. Coli, tetanus, chickenpox, herpes type virus, pin worms, streptothrix (fungi), rabies and altogether over a forty year period, the MOR for about 600 different forms of bacterial and viral forms. The primary frequencies used ranged from the low audio up as high as the limit of short-wave, with several frequencies being combined, and acting both as a carrier as well as a treatment frequency.

Now, this is critical: Rife stated quite clearly that you need the MOR killer frequency of the rod form of the bacillus and the viral form simultaneously to get any effect. Otherwise (his words) you either kill the patient or nothing happens.

This feature is missing from most me-too "Rife machines".

Fortunately, perhaps surprisingly, normal healthy human cells were completely unharmed by these lethal waves.

The MORs for the BX (cancer) and BY (sarcoma) forms of malignancy were listed by Rife as follows:

> 1,604,000
> 11,780,000
> 17,033,663

These are radio frequencies (RF).

By 1935 Rife was ready to begin experiments using his "ray" machine on humans with cancer and TB. Out of 16 terminally ill patients, 14 were pronounced clinically cured after 70 days; the other 2 subsequently recovered after the end of the trial. In other words a 100% success rate on patients in the worst possible condition. This result is outstanding and passes into medical history as a truly great achievement. More shame on those who still refute it, over 70 years later.

THE END

In his career Rife won 14 government awards in recognition of scientific achievements and was honored with a medical degree at the University of Heidelberg in Germany. Yet today his name is often viewed as synonymous with quackery and "Rife machines" are illegal in his home country (though not, of course, elsewhere in the world). That's how far Rife's star has fallen and has yet to be resurrected.

Much has been written about the final destruction of the Rife microscope and "Rife Ray" machines. We have accounts claiming the FDA burst into his office at gun point and smashed all his equipment. The stories of raids are more likely distortions of actions taken against Life Lab Inc, a later company making copycat frequency machines, with Rife as a titular research head but without much involvement (he was scared of further litigation).

It's true that Morris Fishbein, editor of the Journal of the AMA tried to buy into Rife's company Beam Ray and became very maliciously vindictive when he was not allowed to. As a result of his actions doctors using the device were "visited" by the AMA and told to send it back, or face loss of their license (incidentally, Fishbein and the AMA used the same tactics against Harry Hoxsey, who developed a successful herbal cancer cure).

But Rife's own colleagues probably did him nearly as much damage by producing machines which did not stick to the proper specifications and failed to work consistently. Philip Hoyland, the electronics engineer, was paranoid about others stealing the design, which was unpatentable. He tried to disguise the frequencies. Scruples reached a low ebb when a group of British doctors were sold two machines which had been deliberately mis-wired, in order that they could not guess how it worked. They figured it out anyway and, not surprisingly, were very upset at the fraud.

Bertrand Comparet, Rife's lawyer of the time even speculated that Hoyland was sabotaging the program because he desired to grab the action for himself. Hoyland, we know, accepted $10,000 from Fishbein's associates and subsequently was a stooge in their attempt to grab Rife's Beam Ray Corporation. The ensuing litigation was disastrous and although Rife "won" the case, the little company was virtually bankrupt and ceased trading.

A MAN OUT OF TIME

Regardless of all this, I think the final demise of the machine was much simpler to explain and far less dramatic.

Rife came to the market with his machine in the 1930s. It cost $7,000 which in those days was a very considerable investment, even for an MD. No matter, he sold a number.

But also in the 1930s, by a twist of fate, sulfonamide antibiotics swept over the horizon, followed rapidly by penicillin, and this new class of drugs soon overran the therapeutic picture at a fast gallop. When it was possible to knock out virtually any pathogen with a drug costing just a few dollars, quickly, safely and simply (according to perceptions of the day), who would want to invest in a costly machine that was inconveniently large, expensive to run and difficult to operate?

It was the same bad luck with his advanced microscopes. They were the very best of the day, precise and advanced, but very costly. Unfortunately for Rife, the electron microscope was just around the corner (1931) and optical microscopes, no matter how powerful, were doomed to be eclipsed. Of course electron microscopes can only ever look at dead tissue; but that's the fashion in so-called science. Nobody, it seems, wants to do anything so corny as look at real living organisms!

There is another factor little talked about, which is that the authentic Rife machines were super-regenerative RF transmitters. Without going into the technical details, that meant they ultimately fell foul of Federal Communications Commission regulations. Remember, by this time radio stations were springing up all over the US and the FCC devloped strict guidelines as to who was allowed to broadcast, where and at what frequencies. Rife machines were really doomed by this one factor alone.

THE NON-MATERIAL NATURE OF SUBSTANCES

Rife was simply a man out of his time. He died in 1971, frustrated and sad, a broken man, an alcoholic. Most of his knowledge has passed into history and most claims for authentic "Rife machines" are bogus.

In the 1960s a man called John Crane, who had worked with Rife, started selling off the shelf frequency generators as authentic Rife machines; he merely changed the labels on the casing. Crane created the myth that the lower audio frequencies, developed later by Rife and supposed to be used in conjunction with the RF carrier frequencies, were in fact the real MORs.

Clearly this is not true. Recorded MORs are in the far higher RF range. Unfortunately, most modern machines are really derived from Crane, not Rife. Most are even from the same manufacturer, sold under different brand labels. You can tell any of these knock off fakes because they use disease "codes", instead of displaying a frequency.

Don't be fooled by the present Beam Ray Corporation, which is NOT the original Rife company and doesn't have true Rife machines but are simply cashing in on the present interest.

WHAT HAVE WE GOT LEFT?

The real challenge is that, because of the controversy, most modern manufacturers don't want to be known for selling "Rife machines". They use the term frequency generator.

If you want to explore or be part of this technology, choose carefully among the offerings. Let's take one model as an example, the GB-4000. It is made in the USA. Moreover it was designed by a man who has studied and re-created a Rife Ray machine, so at least he knows what he's trying to parallel.

The first good point, is that it uses a frequency band-pass or "sweeping", like the BICOM (p. 101). That means that it will carry out a sweep, passing through a wide range of frequencies.

It has "gating" a surprise new discovery from recent investigations into Rife's old machines, some of which are still around for boffins to pore over. (see below)

It also uses the RF carrier wave method, as well as the lower audio frequencies. It delivers the energy through direct contact (pads and electrodes), so the need for Rife's old-fashioned glass tubes, which generate huge power, are not needed.

THE FUTURE

I'm pleased to report that the blueprint for Rife's wonderful "Universal Microscope" came to light only in the last year. John Marsh had kept it hidden for decades. It will cost a great deal of money to get one built but I for one would donate!

The trouble will be knowing how to use such a complex device.

Also there has been a project to recreate the exact 1939 AZ-58 machine from a schematic given to Crane by John Gruner. So scientifically at least we will have a replica of the technology. One of the surprise discoveries is that the wave form is important; a discontinuous square pulsed wave seems to be the "missing ingredient" from Rife's cook book! This is called "gating".

IT COMES AROUND

Meanwhile, I see that another "breakthrough" was reported in 2007. John Kanzius from Eerie PA claims to have hit on the idea of using radio waves to kill cancer. It sounds remarkably familiar.

Kanzius' idea, in fact, is a little different from Rife's. He proposes sending immunologically tagged nanoparticles to the tumor site (well within current medical science) and then, by bombarding the site with RF, to heat up the tumor and "fry" it (actually called hyperthermia).

Kanzius' idea takes advantage of what Rife found, which is that normal human tissue is transparent to radio frequencies and, in the suggested doses at least, is unharmed by it. In any case the risk of radiation sickness from RF is less than with radiotherapy and far less of a problem than dying of cancer.

I think it will work and work well. It's in trial now. The real question is "Will the cancer industry allow it?"

I don't think so.

CHAPTER 14

BIOLOGY BEYOND DEATH

In chapter 3 the reader will recall I spoke of "biology beyond the skin", meaning that life phenomena are not limited to events taking place inside the body. The whole tenet of this book is that we, as life forms, are not really material in nature but energy and information. The physical form we see is really just an expression of the energy field that is manifested by a yet higher field of information. The correct path to healing therefore is by energetic re-adjustment or, even better, by changing the information field (such as with thought power or psychic energy).

OK, it's been novel and interesting so far; maybe a little challenging in places. Now in this additional chapter for the second edition we come to something truly mind-stretching.

Consider the words "I think the problem is an impedance mismatch into that third transistor in the pre-amp unit... It can be corrected by using a 150 ohm 100 watt resistor in parallel with a 0.0047 microfarad ceramic capacitor..."

Nothing extraordinary about these words. However they were spoken by a man called Dr. George J. Mueller, an electrical engineer who had been dead for 14 years. His speech was captured on an audio tape with a device called a Spiricom by William J. O'Neil, an inventor and electronic technician.

No, I have not lost my mind; I have heard recordings of conversations between O'Neil and Mueller. Dr. Mueller authenticated himself, somewhat, by telling researchers in these post-mortem conversations where to find his birth and death certificate records. He even provided his social security number![1]

If you want to do some authentication yourself, check this pdf file:

http://dspace.library.cornell.edu/bitstream/ 813/3586/ 17/045_
14.pdf [accessed 13th Apr 2008, 2.50 pm PDT]

Mueller also explained intimate details of his life and career at
the University of Wisconsin and Cornell University, which were
later verified*.

In the conversation just referred to, Mueller was helping
O'Neill improve his device for talking with entities from the
world of the dead. It's the weirdest imaginable scenario of a ghost
helping someone Earthside develop their technique for recording
the presence of spectres!

If you miss the point then, truly, the world of wonders we have
is lost on you and I'm sorry.

Well, more of Mueller later. Meanwhile, let's get directly to
grips with the meat of this chapter: electronic communication
with "dead" former life entities. Remember, as we go, that physics tells us that energy cannot be created or destroyed, only transformed. If our living self is indeed an energetic entity, it cannot
go away but only be transformed.

Communication with the dead is not crazy or impossible if
you have a model which makes it realistic. My *Virtual Medicine*
paradigm not only allows for information and energetic entities
but makes it quite clear they MUST be out there, by the laws of
physics. In this exciting new chapter it is my intention to share
abundant evidence that information and energy are superordinate
to matter and that it is our TRUE nature; we are not biochemical
"stuff".

Those who loudly proclaim it is all nonsense or Flim Flam
(James Randi, for instance), are likely to go down in history along
with the pigmy wit of a French scientist, who told his colleagues,
"I have investigated Thomas Edison's phonograph and can assure
you it is nothing more than clever ventriloquism" (a popular
view of the day).

ELECTRONIC VOICE PHENOMENA (EVP)

Face it! "Communicating with the dead" has an automatic dis-
qualifier built in! Those who have engaged deeply in research

into voices captured on electronic devices have preferred the more evasive and less dramatic expression "electronic voice phenomena" or EVP for short. It has a surprising history, unknown to most people.

One of the earliest proponents was none other than Thomas Alva Edison, inventor of the electric light and phonograph. His last major project before his death was building a machine to achieve spirit communication with the dead. His assistant, Dr Miller Hutchinson, wrote, "Edison and I are convinced that in the fields of psychic research will yet be discovered facts that will prove of greater significance to the thinking of the human race than all the inventions we have ever made in the field of electricity."

Edison himself wrote, "If our personality survives, then it is strictly logical or scientific to assume that it retains memory, intellect, other faculties, and knowledge that we acquire on this Earth. Therefore ... if we can evolve an instrument so delicate as to be affected by our personality as it survives in the next life, such an instrument, when made available, ought to record something."[2]

These words show great insight and prescience. Unfortunately, Edison died before he could complete his invention.

In 1936, American photographer Attila von Szalay began experimenting with a record cutter and had moderate success capturing spirit voices on phonograph records. In the 1940s he had better success with the newer but still primitive wire recorder[3].

In 1949, Marcello Bacci of Grosseto, Italy, began experimenting in the paranormal. Soon he began recording voices using an old Nordmende vacuum tube radio. A team of spirits developed around his work, and they spoke to him through the radio sounds. People would visit him in his lab at home, and very often their departed loved ones would talk to them through Mr Bacci's radio.

It is important to observe that Bacci never asked for money or other kinds of financial incentive, which effectively precludes a fraud motive.

In his experiments, Bacci tuned his radio to the short-wave band, in a frequency ranging between 7 and 9 MHz, in a zone clear from normal radio transmissions. After a few minutes the existing background noise disappears and a typical acoustic signal comes out of the loudspeaker, similar to an approaching wind vortex, repeated three or four times at short intervals. Silence then follows, at the end of which an invisible speaker starts to communicate by establishing with Bacci, or with the people attending the experiment, something like a dialogue. Today, Marcello Bacci still uses the vacuum tube radio.[4]

HIS HOLINESS TUNES IN TO THE OTHER SIDE!

In the early 1950s in Italy, two Catholic priests, Father Ernetti and Father Gemelli, were collaborating on music research. Ernetti was an internationally respected scientist, a physicist and philosopher, and also a music lover. Gemelli was President of the Papal Academy. In other words, neither of these guys were flakes.

On September 15, 1952, while Gemelli and Ernetti were recording a Gregorian chant, a wire on their magnetophone kept breaking. Exasperated, Father Gemelli looked up and asked his (deceased) father for help. To the two men's amazement, his father's voice, recorded on the magnetophone, answered, "Of course I shall help you. I'm always with you."

The voice addressed Gemelli as Zucchini. It was a nickname his father had teased him with when he was a boy and no-one else could have known this.

Surprisingly, His Holiness Pope Pius XII in Rome was very accepting and told Gemelli "You really need not worry about this. The existence of this voice is strictly a scientific fact and has nothing whatsoever to do with spiritism. The recorder is totally objective. It receives and records only sound waves from wherever they come. This experiment may perhaps become the cornerstone for a building for scientific studies which will strengthen people's faith in a hereafter." [Gemelli made certain that the experiment did not go public until the last years of his life, so this story wasn't released until 1990][5]

TAPE RECORDINGS

Things started to hot up in 1959, with the work of Swedish film producer Friedrich Juergenson. He first captured voices on audio-tape while taping bird songs. He was startled when he played the tape back and heard a male voice say something about "bird voices in the night." Listening more intently to his tapes, he heard his mother's voice say in German, "Friedrich, you are being watched. Friedel, my little Friedel, can you hear me?"

Juergenson said that when he heard his mother's voice, he was convinced, he had made "an important discovery." During the next four years, Juergenson continued to tape hundreds of paranormal voices. He played the tapes at an international press conference and in 1964 published a book in Swedish: *Voices from the Universe* and then another entitled *Radio Contact with the Dead.*

In 1967, Juergenson's *Radio Contact with the Dead* was translated into German, and Latvian psychologist Dr Konstantin Raudive read it skeptically. He visited Juergenson to learn his methodology, decided to experiment on his own, and soon began developing his own experimental techniques[6]. Like Juergenson, Raudive too heard the voice of his own deceased mother, who called him by his boyhood name: "Kostulit, this is your mother." Eventually he catalogued tens of thousands of voices, many under strict laboratory conditions.

In 1971, the chief engineers of Pye Records Ltd. decided to do a controlled experiment with Konstantin Raudive. They invited him to their sound lab and installed special equipment to block out any radio and television signals. They would not allow Raudive to touch any of the equipment.

Raudive used one tape recorder which was monitored by a control tape recorder. All he could do was speak into a microphone. They taped Raudive's voice for eighteen minutes and none of the experimenters heard any other sounds. But when the scientists played back the tape, to their amazement, they heard over two hundred voices on it.

THE SPIRICOM

The first serious investigators in the US were Paul Jones, George W. Meek and Hans Heckman, who together founded the Metascience Foundation. Their intention from the first was to create a system which would allow two-way voice communication with "The Other Side".

Despite stellar exceptions, as described above, the results from various arrangements of tape recorders, microphones, diodes and radios up to this point had been dogged with several problems. The "voices" were very faint, so that only a person with very acute hearing could detect anything at all. Most of the sounds involved very few words, which raises the likelihood of just coincidental sounds, not true speech. The voices spoke very rapidly (about twice as fast as a typical human being speaks) and often it was difficult to distinguish one word from the next.

Excessive background sound, such as tape hiss, static, white noise, cross talk and equipment hum, added to the difficulty of hearing. To make matters even worse, the shortest phrases would often contain words from two or even three languages (Konstantin Raudive was exceptional in being a multilinguist).

The results of these problems meant that the messages or phrases were so difficult to understand that, if five people were listening, they might have five different opinions as to what was being said.

Not surprisingly, the few parapsychologists who bothered to investigate EVP quickly lost all interest in the subject.

The real breakthrough came when the Metascience Foundation team was joined by a psychically gifted man, William O'Neil, who could not only see and hear spirits, but also knew in-depth electronics. O'Neil recruited several of his spirit friends into the project. One of his invisible colleagues was the spirit of Dr George Jeffries Mueller, already referred to, who simply appeared in O'Neil's living room one day as a semi-materialized spirit, and announced that he was there to assist in the project of Meek and O'Neil.

It became a rather astonishing collaboration with the "dead" Doc Mueller helping Bill O'Neil on Earth design a new piece of electromagnetic equipment that would convert spirit voices into audible voices. Appropriately christened Spiricom, the new device was a set of tone generators and frequency generators that emitted 13 tones spanning the range of the adult male voice.[7]

If you think I have now completely lost contact with reality and reason, let me assure you I have heard Dr Mueller and O'Neil in dialogue myself and am convinced that we have another breakthrough in our understanding of reality. This is totally consistent with my model of *Virtual Medicine* and to me only serves to further underline my view that the Universe is a playground of delights and discoveries. There is so much we don't know and so much yet to discover.

One thing is clear: we survive as energetic and information entities and to repeat my oft-quoted aphorism, advanced physics not only says that it could happen but that it must happen.

THE SPIRIT OF SHARING

One big difference between the attitude of these researchers and the craven self-seeking approach of regular scientists is that they view knowledge as a universal property. Meek and the others have gone out of their way to make all their discoveries public property.

In 1982, G. W. Meek made a trip around the world to distribute tape recordings of 16 excerpts of communications between William J. O'Neil and Mueller. He also distributed a 100-page technical report giving wiring diagrams, photos, technical data and guidelines for research by others.

In the notable words of George Meek, "All researchers affiliated with Metascience Foundation during the ten years of world-wide study of problems and potentials of electronic communication with the so-called "dead" have shared a common goal. They want the fruit of their labors and financial contributions to be made freely available to people of all races all over the world.

"But please note! Everything in the cosmos is energy of one sort or another, and although all energies can be used for good or for evil, it is our hope that the hundreds of individuals and organizations which will carry these developments forward in the decades ahead, will use them ONLY FOR THE GOOD OF ALL MANKIND". [8]

The Foundation did not file any patents in any countries on their many inventions. The name SPIRICOM was never trademarked.

Nevertheless, Meek issues a solemn warning: "If any individuals acting alone or as part of a corporate entity endeavor to use these inventions solely for money-making purposes, or to the detriment of any person, they are herewith forewarned: They should know that the first stop for them, after they sooner or later shed their physical bodies, will be at the bottom of the Lowest Astral Plane".

Oooo!

PHONE CALLS FROM THE OTHER SIDE

If somebody had suggested, decades ago, that I freely accept the idea of dead people contacting the living via telephone, I would have been resistant, I admit.

But in the context of this other irrefutable work in EVP, it's not so hard to believe. In 1979 D. Scott Rogo catalogued them in his book, "Telephone Calls from the Dead."[9]

Possibly the most vivid series of calls were those received from Konstantin Raudive himself. Raudive told several Earthside colleagues that since his death it has been his calling to continue the development of EVP systems from the other side of the veil. He called researcher Mark Macy by phone seven times after his death, and on one occasion the two chatted for nearly 15 minutes before the contact ended.

On another occasion Raudive spoke to Sarah Estep, who had founded the American Association of EVP in 1982. In her shocked surprise, Sarah lapsed to social protocols and said "How are you?" Raudive replied "As well as can be expected for a dead man!"

Is this stretching things too far? Well, why not information systems over the phone (non-local)? Albert Abrams stumbled across it in 1922, remember (p. 9). Time and again it comes back to this man of genius and vision.

COMPUTERS TOO, OBVIOUSLY

How many of us have been convinced at times that our computer was infected with some kind of demonic life energy that keeps losing files and corrupting data? Well, maybe it was literally true.

Take the case of English school teacher Ken Webster and his haunted computer. Beginning in the Autumn of 1984, a series of poltergeist events took place, focused on the kitchen area, including the stacking of objects, noises, marks on the walls and `thrown' objects. What made this visitation different was the appearance of messages on a word processor.

Personal computers were only just appearing in 1984 and, as a school teacher, Webster had borrowed a primitive BBC `B' computer from school. These machines had around 32k of memory, a word processor on an installed chip and the only means of saving files was to a floppy disk on an external drive. No networking, no modem, definitely no Internet.

One evening, the computer was accidentally left on and when Webster and his girlfriend Debbie returned there was a `message', a poem of sorts. It was treated as a joke of course, but saved to disk anyway.

A different machine was borrowed on another occasion and another inexplicable communication was received.

This time the language had an archaic flavour, seemingly of Elizabethan English. The tone of this second message was threatening and Webster felt the joke was now in bad taste.

In an attempt to catch the obvious hoaxer, yet another computer was brought home. Its disc was examined for preloaded material (there was little software in those days, in any case; hackers and other geeks were a long way into the future). Webster and his girlfriend checked the locks on the house and left the computer running in the kitchen. Another message appeared in the same quirky 'mock Tudor' style.

Webster decided to type in a reply and, astonishingly, this was met with a further response. Two-way communications began in earnest with a male entity who declared himself to be one Tomas Harden, which lasted over a period of sixteen months.

Various investigators have offered no enable explanation (beyond a true electronic incarnation). But Debbie Oakes, Webster's girlfriend, seems pivotal. Neither the mysterious moving objects or cyber messages from "beyond" occurred unless she was in the vicinity.

Time and again I have learned that discarnate entities need the energies of others in order to "perform" their tricks. Poltergiest activity is known to be a telekinetic effect that surrounds one particular person (usually undergoing some kind of emotional turmoil). Maybe she was the fuel tank of this computer ghost?

Given the primitive standard of the hardware, it is not possible to offer as an explanation that these computers were capable of developing AI. So maybe the presence in the machine was none other than Mr. Tomas Harden, deceased. Was he angry at the couple for occupying his house? Or lasciviously inclined towards Ms Debbie Oakes?

The whole story is told in Webster's book, now out of print and selling for black market prices: *The Vertical Plane,* Grafton, London 1989.[10]

The manifestation of an apparently ancient spirit in modern guise seems remarkably similar to another computer possession story. Reverend Jim Peasboro, from Savannah, GA not only believes in computers being possessed by evil energies – he has written a book about it entitled The Devil in the Machine. According to him, today's thinking machines have enough space on their hard drives to accommodate Satan or one of his cronies. "Any PC built after 1985 has the storage capacity to house an evil spirit," the minister confirmed.

Don't laugh.

Whereas I respectfully submit that Peasboro's obsession with Lucifer has more to do with his own world view, I see no reason, in the light of many other examples of contact we are sharing here, to doubt that some kind of malicious energy was seeking a confrontation with this man of the Church.

On the day in question Peasboro was sitting at the keyboard of one of his parishioners, investigating the possibility of a possession, when to his surprise, an artificial-intelligence program fired up -- without him clicking it on. Then according to the reverend's testimony, the machine began mocking him by typing out the words 'Preacher, you are a weakling and your God is a damn liar.' After that the device went haywire and started printing out what appeared to be gobbledygook.

"I later had an expert in dead languages examine the text," the minister said. "It turned out to be a stream of obscenities written in a 2,800-year-old Mesopotamian dialect!"[11]

KURT CURBAIN LIVES!

A 24-year-old bar manager from Essex, England became perturbed when her Compaq laptop seemed to take in the ghost of deceased rock star Kurt Cobain. His ghostly image would appear on screen and demand she give him a kiss. The strange thing was this only ever happened after the computer was switched off. The owner was, not surprisingly, rather unnerved and confessed, "I'm not a spiritual person...I had to do something."

So she arranged a computer exorcism. It worked. The ghost has never been since. Unfortunately, the computer then refused to work at all. Excess holy water was blamed. But it seems to me the living energy entity in the machine has had the last laugh.

VOICES ON RADIO

There have been well documented instances of strange apparitional voices coming over on radio and TV. I remember one startling occasion when it happened while I was watching TV. The BBC, I remember, apologized for the "technical hitch". These are naturally dismissed as quirks of the ionosphere that somehow result in distant channels breaking into the local broadcast (the UFO people, predictably, think it's aliens trying to make contact from craft hovering near the Earth).

Probably intrusive transmissions do happen. But I believe that many instances of genuine communication are being lost because nobody is thinking along EVP lines. It's almost automatic to dismiss such events as a technical anomaly and not even consider other possibilities.

Let me share a historical and well-documented contact which defies science. The Dawkins and other rigid conventional scientists can only fall back on trite explanations like "mass hysteria" and "technical glitch" (since their world will not admit the obvious simple explanation: that these events actually occurred in the terms described).

In 1983 Hans Otto Koenig appeared on a popular radio program on Europe's largest radio station, Radio Luxembourg, featuring his extremely low frequency oscillators, with lights in the ultraviolet and infrared range. The program host, Rainer Holbe, had Koenig set up his equipment under close supervision of the station engineers. One of the engineers asked if a voice could come through in direct reply to a question, and a discarnate voice quickly replied over the system, "We hear your voice. Otto Koenig makes wireless contact with the dead."

Stunned, Rainer Holbe addressed the millions of listeners across Europe, "I tell you, dear listeners of Radio Luxembourg, and I swear by the life of my children, that nothing has been manipulated. There are no tricks. It is a voice, and we do not know from where it comes." The station issued an official statement afterwards. Every step of the program was carefully supervised. Staff and engineers were convinced that the voices were paranormal.

Numerous other experiments with radio have had similar success, inexplicable in any other simple terms than contact from other planes of consciousness.

FINALLY, VIDEO FROM "THE OTHER SIDE"!

Well, why not? Given that discarnate beings can leave audio traces on a magnetic tape, why not images on a VCR?

Klaus Schreiber began to receive spirit images on his TV set in 1985, including the faces of scientist Albert Einstein, Austrian actress Romy Schneider, and various departed family members, especially his two deceased wives and daughter Karin, with whom he was particularly close. I have seen these recordings and can assure readers they are not artefactual or just "interpretations". I wasn't sure about the Einstein likeness; all I will admit is, it looked very like him.

The technique here is rather special. It involves pointing a video camera at a television monitor, which is playing the image captured by the camera. So the camera records its own output; a kind of feedback loop. This is so like the foundation of fractals and Ludwig van Bertalanffy's natural living "systems" that I concede its plausibility right away.

What happens is that the swirling cloud of energies captured on screen gradually resolves into a recognizable image. Sometimes these move; sometimes the eyes or mouth of the "ghost" image will open or close. It's very eerie to watch.

Maggy Harsch-Fischbach and her husband Jules Harsch of Luxembourg began to get spectacular voice contacts through radio systems early in their experiments in 1985. A high-pitched, computer-like voice came through their radios with growing frequency to share amazing insights with the couple.

The voice identified itself as a conscious entity which was never human, never animal, and never in a physical body. "I am not energy and I am not a light being. You are familiar with the picture of two children walking across a bridge, and behind them is a being who protects them. That's what I am to you, but without the wings. You can call me Technician, since that is my role in opening up this communication bridge. I am assigned to Planet Earth."

He lived up to his promise.

The small apartment inhabited by the Harsch-Fischbachs became a place of astounding manifestations, as visiting scientists and reporters from all over the world saw spirit images flash across the TV screen and heard long discourses by various deceased personalities through radio sounds. The spirit of Nelson D. Rockefeller told German physicist Ernst Senkowski, "The Mahatmas are a reality."

Nineteenth-Century chemist Henri Ste. Claire de Ville appeared and told American and German researchers, "It is our job as well as your job to set fire to minds—to set fire to minds in your world, and in that moment to try to master time."

Fritz Malkhoff and Adolf Homes began EVP experiments independently in 1987, and each began to get spirit voices on tape rather quickly. In a few months, they learned of each other's work, and they became colleagues and friends. During their experiments, small voices on radio quickly developed long, clear voices.

Then they began to receive phone calls from spirits, and in 1988 they set up Malkhoff's computer in the house of Adolf Homes, where they did most of their experiments. They posed a short question, and two days later a short answer appeared miraculously on their computer screen.

THE OLD TIMERS COME AROUND AGAIN!

Homes received spirit images on his television and messages on his computer screen rather routinely. One morning in 1994, Homes climbed out of bed in a trance, aimed a video camera at his television, and received the first color picture from the spirit worlds. It was a picture of deceased EVP pioneer Friedrich Juergenson.

At the same time, a message from Juergenson printed out on Homes's computer, stating, "This is Friedel from Sweden. I am sending you a self-portrait... The projection since January 17, 1991, has been in the quantum of spacelessness and timelessness. All your and our thoughts have their own electromagnetic reality which does not get lost outside the space-time structure... Consciousness creates all form...."

In other words, Juergensen seems to be reassuring us that we do, as physics predicts, survive as an electromagnetic reality.

This of course says nothing about the true nature of the soul and I have no wish here to intrude on the beliefs of any reader or group.

Where is all this leading? Well, one of the fascinating developments is that the first generation of pioneers, as they aged and died, have started to come back through EVP systems and continue their work from the "other" perspective!

MARK MACY AND INIT

In 1995, Macy went on to join with other researchers and found INIT, the International Network for Instrumental Transcommunication. At the same time EVP took on a new label: ITC or instrumental transcommunication.

INIT members report regular and helpful contact from spirit friends. The most inspiring and helpful information came from a group of timeless beings who said they had never been in physical bodies, but had observed human development over many thousands of years.

This group of entities told INIT on more than one occasion that simply opening the door to the spirit worlds can be dangerous, but researchers who work together and dedicate their efforts to higher human principles will receive ethereal guidance and protection.

As years passed, Technician and his six ethereal friends, along with a team of more than 1,000 spirit beings who had once lived on Earth, shared vast and astonishing information with INIT members through computers, telephones, radios, and other technical media. The ethereal beings said they had accompanied our world for many thousands of years and had come close six times when the Earth had reached a crossroads leading either to a dark age or to a period of enlightenment.

This, they said, was the seventh time, and they wished to establish a lasting bridge between Earth and their formless realm of wise, loving consciousness. ITC research would be the means by which to establish that bridge.

That being so, I would suggest that this chapter covers matters of grave importance to us all.

ON A DARKER NOTE

INIT was told that contact with spirits are made possible by a "contact field", which is a pool of thoughts and attitudes of all researchers collaborating on an ITC project. When the thoughts and attitudes of all those entities on both sides of the veil are in harmony, the contact field was clear. The discarnate entities could then see into our world and work with our equipment.

When doubts, fears, envy, resentment, and other troubled feelings created dissonance, the contact field becomes cloudy.

Unfortunately, that's what happened to INIT. After several years, troubles developed. Some members began working with scientists in their home country, who predictably dismissed the validity of this research. The "scientists" told the INIT members they should be more skeptical of the contacts their colleagues were reporting. So some members began to express doubts publicly about the legitimacy of other members' contacts. There were shocks and betrayals, leading to breakdown of camaraderie.

As a result of the dissent, the contact field became cloudy, and the miracles of ITC virtually dried up. Mark Macy reports that messages of great depth and import have not been reported from any researchers since the year 2000, to the best of his knowledge.

Nowadays the American Association of Voice Phenomena has taken over center stage (http://www.aaevp.com). There is even an initiative to establish "best practices" in EVP. That page was last modified just before this book went to press, 01:16, 8 April 2008.

DO YOU WANT TO TRY?

Anybody can do this. It could be your first real reach into dimensions beyond this one. It's certainly a novel way to surf reality! I've extracted the following beginner's advice from Mark Macy's website at www.worlditc.org

First, says Macy, when conducting EVP experiments, take a sober, serious approach and focus on the positive. Experiment only when you're in a happy, enthusiastic, unfettered frame of mind.

Use an audiocassette recorder with an external microphone and a source of mild white noise (such as a radio tuned between stations). Place the microphone a few feet from the radio. Turn on the tape recorder and introduce the session.

Name the date and time and ask a few short questions, then replay the sequence and listen closely. A set of earphones can help make the short, faint voices more audible.

Some people get voices on their very first try; others work for months before getting their first voice. Konstantin Raudive experimented diligently for three months before getting his first voice. Yet he went on to record, analyze and collect more than 70,000 voices, many under strict laboratory conditions.

EVP researchers all agree you must conduct voice experiments on a regular basis. In that way you grow your "contact field" and the voices will become louder and clearer. Always remember, as I said about the EAV machines (chapter 5, the psychokinetic effect), you are part of the equipment.

This isn't a matter of building self-delusion. Other people can hear the voices quite clearly too, when the recordings are good.

BE WARNED: Entities may occasionally menace researchers and perhaps announce that the experimenter will have bad experiences very soon. Troubled voices sometimes predict illness for the experimenter, relatives or friends, and even death. Words of hate and pessimism, destruction and violence can sometimes be heard.

My own belief is that screwed up and out of balance entities are no more powerful than everyday inept and dysfunctional humans. They can accomplish nothing, unless you react with a negative state of mind and concede your own power to them.

The only possible danger arises if you yourself take it on board, like a suggestible hypnotic subject. Therefore do not enter this communication domain if you do not have a point of balance. You need to be strongly centered within your own energetic being.

BETTER EQUIPMENT
As you get more experienced, you can consider technical improvements.

Germanium diode.
Konstantin Raudive himself devised a way to improve EVP voices with a germanium diode instead of a microphone connected to the audio input of a standard tape recorder. Solder a 1N914 germanium diode (available from Radio Shack) to a jack, or male plug, that will fit the microphone input of your tape recorder. Plug this modified jack into the recorder, turn the volume up all the way, and start recording. With this setup, the recorder will

not record human voices nor other normal sounds in the room; just spirit voices.

Radios.

Discarnate voices have intellect and information but lack energy. They have to parasitize existing energy.

You can provide that, using white noise ("static") between channels on a radio tuner. In fact I have been told that at a pinch you can use the sound of running water. Since learning that, many transcendental poetic experiences near flowing streams and the sea have suddenly made sense to me!

Spirit voices apparently find it easier to create their voice from existing voice fragments than to fashion one out of blank white noise. So tuning in to foreign-language broadcasts is a good idea, it makes it easier to distinguish between the radio noises and possible spirit voices you receive in your language.

Again, at a pinch, operators can simply talk inconsequentially to each other and then play back the recording, listening for superimposed voices.

Reel-to-Reel Tape recorders.

Some people claim to get better results with a reel-to-reel tape recorder than with the more common cassette recorder. On cassette recorders it's good to have a "cue" or "review" function so that while the recorder is in "play" mode you can press down a bit on the "reverse" or "fast forward" button to move quickly a few inches backward or forward on the tape, then resume playing simply by releasing the "reverse" or "fast forward" button. Make sure it has a rev counter.

Computers.

Some voice experimenters today are using computers with attached microphones instead of tape recorders. Advantages of the computer, says Macy, include clarity of the voices, immediate playback, reproduction without loss of quality, and easy transportability of sound files to the internet. The drawback of computers is the fact that voice files take up a lot of memory.

Digital Pocket Recorders

That last word in EVP technology, apparently, is the Sony ICD B7 digital pocket recorder. I got mine for only $50, so the cost of getting involved is not high!

WHAT HAS ALL THIS TO DO WITH VIRTUAL MEDICINE?

You may think I have spent too long on a curious byway in knowledge. Ghosts and discarnate beings tell us more about the nature of life itself but nothing about healing.

I disagree. One of the common themes I meet in my contact with many peoples and races in connection with my profession is that of "spirit helpers". Remarkable psychic healings have been achieved, that defy all scientific rationale. Often the gifted individuals who are capable of these miracles of recovery speak of other presences, perhaps with more power than they have alone, and which aided the recovery (I almost wrote recovery process but these events seem to me more like transformations than mere recovery through process). Those who have been healed sometimes report the sensation of several pairs of hands working on their body.

I have not introduced this dimension before but on reviewing the work for the second edition I think it is only right that this element is now considered, because of the technological nature of these apparitions. They are "virtual beings" come to us in an electromagnetic energy format. Their role in healing may soon become apparent and I for one would like to help birth it.

We have seen from their comments that deceased entities are willing to work with us in evolving better functioning communications equipment. Well, why not better healing devices and procedures? It's probably already happening but largely unrecognized.

I have in mind startling developments such as the Vo-Cal 360 voice re-patterning machine. The inventor Calvin Young has told us that he often had a sense of being guided by beings from a higher consciousness in what steps to take to evolve his breakthrough technology. Moreover, those of us who use it have often encountered "presences", such as a dead ancestor, appearing as an energy manifestation and assisting in the healing process or being healed, during the V-Cal procedure.

Who knows: Royal Raymond Rife may show up and tell us more about his amazing technical system for healing. I hope so!

In keeping with the forward-looking theme of these final chapters, I would like to suggest that it may be the next big direction we go to in health sciences and healing devices.

In fact conscious discarnate entities may already be controlling the information output of devices like the MORA machine and so-called "conscious interface" devices (EPFX, SCIO and similar). This will explain the anomaly I have called attention to for years, which is that many people cannot make these latter devices work. That should not be if the scientific pretensions of the inventor were correct.

But it makes sense if discorporate entities are the real heart work of the machine and not the suspect software. That would still please many of Bill Nelson's followers and discomfit only a few, I suspect.

Those operators who were successful either had systems which came with a ready and willing entity from a higher level. Or the operator was a sensitive, capable of developing rapport with such a being and tapping into its deep knowledge and awareness. This would explain many of the almost miraculous case interventions and the resultant recoveries.

Last Word, In Every Sense

Let me leave the closing words of this chapter to long-dead Swedish film producer Friedrich Juergenson. He told eager experimenters in Germany, watching through the television of Adolf Homes, "Every being is a unity of spirit and body that cannot be separated on Earth or in spirit. The only difference is the fact that the physical body disintegrates and in its place comes the astral body.

"Our message [from this side] is to tell you that your life goes on. Any speculations on how an individual will experience it are bound to be limited in accuracy. All your scientific, medical or biological speculations miss the mark of these realities. What serves as 'real' to science is not close to reality in the broad picture. It is no more than a word in a book."

I couldn't agree more.

CHAPTER 15
ELECTRONIC KUNDALINI

A view of the new medical paradigm I have called VIRTUAL MEDICINE would be incomplete without looking at the deeper philosophical implications of what this new domain of knowledge is teaching us. Few doctors to date are even fully aware of the progress that has been made in this field, much less espoused the system of healing it engenders. But nevertheless, there is a clear situation where advances in healing science and technology, such as I described in the last chapter, have led us to a new appreciation of the very meaning of life.

Life is no longer merely the flesh. We 'live' outside the skin! To me these new horizons are significant, since it is largely a doctor's role to be expert in these matters and be able to inform the public about the issues. This seems to me to have been majorly lacking in recent times. Probably this is one of the reasons why so-called alternative medicine has become prominent. If members of the medical profession will not fulfil the role for which patients feel a yearning, then it is open to others to fill the gap.

I have always felt that the real meaning of healing and 'doctoring' was to be able to see the patient in the wider context as a life form in a big brawling universe and to seek to bring healing at this level. Only to remove or suppress symptoms is really to miss most of the problem, which is that the patient is out of balance and is experiencing a degree of separation from their true place in the cosmos. In this view, disease is just the result of this lack of integration leading to dis-ease.

The traditional shamanic healer knows far more about man's true nature and our place in the scheme of things than a scientifically trained Western 'medicine man'. They understand healing at what I deem to be a far deeper level of awareness than science.

The Hollywood cliché portrayal of the witch-doctor as an ignorant savage who is marginalized by a hero who steps in with a life-
saving penicillin shot has always seemed to me to be completely
backwards. The fact is that more people on earth get well more of
the time by using the safe and traditional healing approach than
get well by means of drugs. The trouble is that doctors see too
many such movies and start to believe their own propaganda.

And it is only propaganda. There is much to be ashamed of
in the way modern medicine is conducted. The manner of arrogantly over-riding simple human values of love, trust, honesty
and humility is one such embarrassment. I have been involved
in many shamanic experiments and can assure the reader that
a dramatic 'soul-retrieval' as it is called has often been effective in a cure, where conventional medicine was simply unable
to help. That's just one of those things, you may suppose. But
what nobody needs is the profession which failed to help, scoff-
ing and deriding the one which did! There's no true science in
these childish shows of pique and it does not serve the cause of
genuine enquiry.

In that sense this book is offered as a small light in the new
dawn of which it is but a tiny part. It was also written in the
hope that, by sticking fairly close to the scientific model, it will
partly persuade those who think otherwise that there are many
strange and vital manifestations of life which are not merely illu-
sions. In fact, using the equipment I have described in the previous chapters, one cannot fail to be impressed by the obviousness
of mysterious forces that interplay with our lives and give it far
more meaning than just the foraging and procreation of a carbon
dioxide engine.

I have found these devices to be not merely diagnostic tools
but they are in a sense learning systems. If only medical students
were shown some of the properties of tissue and pathogens that
are seen clearly when practising VIRTUAL MEDICINE it would
give them a totally different orientation in their chosen profession. They would gain respect for the divine, the supernormal
and the simply awesome characteristics of nature and life. To see
how the human energies kick over when a pathogen is merely

brought close to the body (but not touching it) I always feel is to teach us something about ourselves and our true nature, not just the mechanism of disease.

The well-trained doctor of the future may begin to talk a little bit like the shamans or magicians of old, there the central role of manifest reality and the conscious interaction with it is the sole and total basis of life renewal and healing forces. I don't think that means we will never use antibiotics, anaesthetics, lasers or the other paraphernalia of modern high-tech medicine. But I hope that, through time, the adoption of the techniques and (even more importantly) the principles outlined in this book will become the mainstay of medical practise. I fervently believe that technological medicine now finds itself at a watershed. It is a time of a collective paradigm shift, when professional and scientific attitudes move from one set of truths to another.

STICKING WITH SCIENCE

It has been the purpose of this text all through to avoid everything that is New Age sugar cake and concentrate on objective facts, albeit novel ones. This is for a very good reason; it is necessary to de mystify these life phenomena and get rid of the silliness and supposition that science is somehow 'wicked' and that everything that matters and is nourishing in healing is somehow superior, other worldly (even 'divine') and forever beyond Man's ken. This mystical and fairy story rhetoric is proving a serious barrier to wider acceptance of this knowledge by the scientific and medical community.

It would be more tolerable if the some of the hands on alternative practitioners who profess to manipulate energies were more willing to subject their favourite methods to the same kind of rigorous testing scrutiny that scientists are required to do. The discipline would blow away quite a few cobwebs, open doors and start to build bridges of respect from one movement to the other.

As Dr. Julian Kenyon, co founder of The Centre for the Study of Complementary Therapies in Southampton, UK, has stated: 'The idea of applying scientific measurement to energetic parameters has not been greeted with enthusiasm by the often doctrinaire proponents of skills such as traditional Chinese medicine and classical homeopathy in particular. Many of these disciplines are surrounded by some degree of mystique, a proportion of which does not stand up to critical examination'.

It might be assumed that I am taking a position here which does not believe in the divine manifestation of life or that there is nothing beyond physics, nothing we can call the soul or spirit, no God or no ineffable quality of it all.

Not so. Indeed, the opposite is true. I care passionately about the life immortal and the nature of what may be termed 'transcendental'. I have spent years researching past lives, discarnate entities, soul retrieval and similar phenomena as part of healing.

KEY QUESTION

One of the key questions which will have suggested itself to the reader (especially in the last chapter) is: 'Where does the boundary of theoretical physics end and where does the transcendental or consciousness mystery begin?' In fact one can extend this question and ask 'Is it a sharp boundary or is there a gradual blurring from ordinary reality to the super-normal or metaphysical?'. One would also be justified in wondering if the threshold actually moves and, if so, under what circumstances? Or is it perhaps always fixed and a matter of divine construct?' These are meaty questions but it seems to me that those of us at the cutting edge should be asking them. The time is right for that 'quantum shift' into the Age of Aquarian consciousness, which may be our gift to the coming generations, as much as the Renaissance was to those from the fourteenth century onwards. I do not know the answer to any of the boundary questions; but just to ask them and appreciate their significance is intellectually stimulating.

Is our world the property of our consciousness, or the other way round?

So much of what is detected by these strange new medical devices rests on subtle perceptions that one is justified in believing that the mind actually plays a part in the process which is taking place at the diagnostic interface. Most of these devices are not absolute detectors, in the precise sense that a blood test or an x-ray radiograph is. The individual practitioner influences the results considerably by his or her understanding and knowledge system; we have seen that there is an inevitable energy input also. Any two individuals who stand together unconsciously and inescapably pool their energy resources into a common resultant field. This is where the placebo effect comes from; it is implicit in all medicine.

Far from making VIRTUAL MEDICINE unscientific, it means that we share some of the interpretation difficulties of modern physics. Indeed Niels Bohr's extreme view of quantum mechanics, the so-called 'Copenhagen Interpretation' (Bohr was Danish), is that one cannot detach objectivity from the measurer. There simply is no means of contacting the objective, even if such a thing were to actually exist, so we may as well forget about it. There is something there but as soon as you look at it, it changes and becomes a merely subjective encounter.

Some scientists are beginning to speak of "subjective reality" as if it were a given.

CHILDHOOD'S END

A better idea is to come to terms with this 'limitation' and see it instead, as some of us do, as a wide wonderful new indicator towards something greater and as yet not fully seen. And I include in this man's religions. It is not conceited to aver that perhaps we have only just begun to expand our awareness to the point where we can begin to move out into the bigger cosmos. It may be that what we have clung to as religion thus far is nothing more than childish metaphors for a nascent reality that has been dimly perceived and yet just beyond our grasp.

We need to think again about consciousness and use it to reframe science. I would like to see a friendlier gentler science which recognizes that the properties of the physical universe (physics) are the same as those of the mind. Indeed, as long ago as 1911 the now beloved 11th edition of ENCYCLOPAEDIA BRI-

TANNICA [http://www.1911encyclopedia.org] stated plainly that space and time have no meaning outside the mind and that these two elements of reality would only be understood when the mind's role in manifesting them became known.

If this comes about then we can stop thinking of ourselves as lowly admirers of a vast and almost incomprehensible cosmos but take our place as part of the very process of creation. Far from being overwhelmingly large, it becomes a testimony, a statement of the power of consciousness and the immanent, ineffable qualities of our Being.

Then physics starts to sound like religion, as Buddhism had always seemed to me to sound rather like a mixture of psychology and physics.

This blurring of the boundary between the properties mind and theoretical physics was the theme of a general public wake up in the late 1970s, occasioned by popular texts such as *The Dancing Wu Lei Masters* by Gary Zukov and *The Tao of Physics* by Fritjof Capra. Both authors brought together the existing knowledge in the mysterious world of quantum physics and showed how closely our present understanding of the supposedly objective and 'real' world paralleled the postulated creation of existence described long ago in the Sanscrit Vedas and the Pali canon. One was indeed impressed by the striking convergence of two (apparently) alien intellectual streams.

It was, as I said earlier in the present text, a matter of science catching up with esoteric wisdom, rather than the other way round. I think Einstein's metaphor is even more apposite:

'....creating a new theory is not like destroying an old barn and erecting a skyscraper in its place. It is rather like climbing a mountain, gaining new and wider views, discovering unexpected connections between our starting point and its rich environment. But the point from which we started out still exists and can be seen, although it appears smaller and forms a tiny part of our broad view gained by the mastery of the obstacles on our adventurous way up'.

WESTERN ENERGY MEDICINE

One of my pet hobby horses is the nature of emerging Western energy medicine. Contrary to what many people think, I do not believe it will be a watery make over of the Chinese, Vedic, or similar models.

We have our own contribution to make and that is in the dazzling field of technology. I have shared with the reader many devices which are so far out to the perimeter of our knowledge that they seem almost magical.

But then the late Arthur C. Clark is famous for saying "Any technology which is sufficiently advance is indistinguishable from magic".

This was the third of three laws by him. The first, "When a distinguished but elderly scientist states that something is possible, he is almost certainly right. When he states that something is impossible, he is very probably wrong" was proposed by Clarke in the essay "Hazards of Prophecy: The Failure of Imagination", in Profiles of the Future (1962).

The second law is offered as a simple observation in the same essay: "The only way of discovering the limits of the possible is to venture a little way past them into the impossible". Its status as Clarke's Second Law was conferred on it by others.

The third law appeared in a 1973 revision of Profiles of the Future, Clarke acknowledged the Second Law and proposed the Third in order to round out the number, adding "As three laws were good enough for Newton, I have modestly decided to stop there."

On this theme, let me add a re-writing of another "law" which may be relevant to the criticisms of my Virtual Medicine model: The eminence of a famous figure in science can be measured by how long he holds back progress in his field.

THE PICTURE

I see that Western energy medicine may soon give us electro-magnetically encoded medicines, instead of the real thing (will there be side-effects from this virtual medicine?)

We may also consider encoded remedies of all kinds and why not nutritional supplements? (I would always recommend that the patient takes areal supplement too).

Then there is the electromagnetic disruption or zapping of cancer cells and pathogens (nuking, as youngsters would say) in the Rife frequency generator model (chapter 13).

We have detection of electromagnetic signatures of disease well under control in the EAV and cyclotron resonance model.

I don't think it is far from now that the time will come when, if a child or adult is sick, it will be possible to slip a disc into the computer which will diagnose the disease; then we click the button which says "Heal" (followed by a pop up which asks "Are you sure you want to heal?" Of course!)

The system then plays soothing and healing frequencies which eliminate the real cause of the disease, re-establish harmony and promote fast, effective healing.

In fact I would say it's very close.

THOUGHT MACHINES

One of science's fashions is to chase the grail of computers which can think like humans. The so-called Turing Test, named after British mathematician Alan Turing, is supposed to define the moment at which a machine can actually 'think' or at least appear to think by fooling the observers.

Another more important search is under way, a kind of electronic holism and, so far, Big Business is leaving it to those who care. We may soon have machines which embody REAL human thought, in other words machines which are a composite of physical matter and human mind.

The fact is, the horizon between consciousness and physical reality is fast becoming so blurred I predict that within the first twenty years of this millennium we will have computers which can interact directly with thought.

It will depend on two directions of progress: expanding our consciousness, making it more intensely coherent, and the development of small scale electronics which are capable of sensing changes in our thought processes.

Both prerequisites are well advanced.

Boffins and engineers have attempted to expand the physical limitations of computing, trying to devise new ways to get more and more computing power using less and less physical resources. Electronics hardware systems have shrunk by half approximately every 18 months in the past twenty years. If this trend continues, soon individual electronic logic gates (the decision points that once upon a time were clumsy transistors) will be down to the size of atoms and currents will be measured in terms of the number of electrons which move. There is no theoretical reason this cannot come about; it is merely a question of the present technical difficulties.

The problem is that, when computer systems are so small, reliability reaches its practical limit. Nano-electronics operations become subject to disruption by 'noise' or extraneous interference. There are surprising new sources of such noise, including mysterious alpha particle 'pollution' from unknown sources, which continue to challenge the limitations of practical physics.

It seems likely the human thought processes can also become 'noise' and disrupt computations. We have already seen from chapter 1 that the brain and mind processes can give off magnetic fields detectable by SQUIDs. It is only a matter of time before this effect is harnessed and deliberate connection of thought energy processes to a computer becomes a reliable reality.

It must happen eventually, since even non-material conscious entities can partly influence electronic apparatus, as we saw in chapter 14.

KUNDALINI AWAKENING

How can we seek to strengthen our consciousness and what criteria evince any improvement? Historically, our Western culture has viewed consciousness in the same order of reference as intelligence. The supposition is that more mental power means more storage and retrieval from contents of a warehouse or database somewhere within the mind. It is a computer-oriented view and is fine as far as it goes.

But it has nothing whatever to do with consciousness. The very same comparison with computers proves the point: to have a massive memory and algorithmic capability does not imply any awareness of the process going on in one's silicon guts.

Gradually we are being forced to look at a more holistic paradigm, for the psyche and for reality. The new model of consciousness is one of information or constructive input into experience: subject-dependent reality (no "absolute" reality) and formative causation (created, not merely observed, reality).

I could not presume to define consciousness but I think I am not exactly out on a limb in saying that it clearly implies some participative interaction with reality. It is about the ACTUAL experience and not the logging or recording of experience, as in the cyber domain. In other words it centres around perception and not memory.

Thus anything which increases perception ability is valid material with which to expand consciousness.

Traditional Eastern meditative practices have always utilized a rather passive and dissociative aim in relation to developing finer consciousness. The assumption is that by quieting the 'chatter' within the mind, the greater consciousness will emerge, rather like a timid fawn creeping out of the forest where it has hidden. Isolation tank research has tended to support this view, where 'less' means 'more'. Subjects describe inspired new levels of perception and feeling when once the noise within falls silent. Biofeedback techniques also seem to work better when the subject gives up trying and just relaxes in expectation.

There are two main problems with this traditional passive approach: it takes too long and it does not focus with coherence sufficient to be likely to waken up an electronics system. Some newer approach is required. Interesting new possibilities are emerging all the time.

PSYCHOKINESIS

Psychic effects at a distance are known as PK or psychokinesis. These have been shown to take place, I think without any doubt. We need urgently to understand how. It seems to be telling us that the human mind, computationally and behaviourally, must exist separately from the physical brain (*). For those of us who have been outside the body, there can be no other view.

The necessary mind-brain link probably comes within known physics laws but that at present it remains hidden from view simply because of current practical limitations and gaps in our theoretical understanding (as was the case for so many centuries with the body's energy field). All we can say with our present state of knowledge is that a thought potential somehow excites an electro-magnetic response which can then act at a distance and create the desired effect.

Once the electro-magnetic field is involved, there is no real mystery to effects at a distance. We have already seen that the human energy field can damage or disrupt computers, watches and other sensitive electronic equipment. I wrote about it in *The Allergy Handbook* and suggested that allergy sufferers seemed to have a far more powerful electro-magnetic 'aura' than most people. As a spectacular demonstration of this human energy charge, an experiment was conducted at the Menninger Foundation. Exceptional subject were suspended in front of a large wired copper wall and were shown to give off very substantial electro-magnetic fields, easily capable of disrupting micro-electronics.

But these psychic effects still trouble the hard-line mechanistic scientists, who get so inflamed with anything that implies vitalism that they would prefer to dismiss evidence as hallucination, rather than rethink any part of their precious model. This narrowness is hardly in accord with the principles of seeking the WHOLE truth. However I am pleased to report that a number of keen thinkers are no longer satisfied to dismiss metaphysics in this way: they would rather refresh and stretch the boundaries of physics, so that what is observed is no longer 'meta'!

A cadre of scientists have taken the view that if quantum theory is the best explanation of reality we have at present, then it should take account of mind and consciousness. Quantum theory cannot be considered independently of the observer effect, which tells us that observation of the physical system in question will instantaneously alter its state at all points of reference. Note that 'instantaneous' means faster than the speed of light, which is not allowed in relativity but sits comfortably with observations in the quantum domain.

QUANTUM CONSCIOUSNESS

Professor D F Lawden at Aston University, Birmingham, UK, is among those who think that systems which are dependent on the observer state, that is which include consciousness in the nature of the construct, are especially worthy of study. The VIRTUAL MEDICINE diagnostic and therapeutic techniques I have detailed in this book are just such examples of psycho-physical states displaying quantum characteristics.

Lawson has gone so far as to draw up modifications of the basic equations of quantum mechanics, to allow for possible disturbing psychic effects being introduced by the participants. This has also helped to clarify what constraints to 'reality' there may be, when recognizing there is no absolute or autonomous state. In this, Lawden likens quantum science to the philosophy of George Berkeley, one of the three principal British Empiricist philosophers (along with David Hume and John Locke).

It is no exaggeration to say that this revision effectively turns science on its head (Dawkins take note) and puts ideas and sensations as the primary events, and matter (particles, energy) as secondary participants; this is exactly where our eastern forebears left our cosmos four thousand years ago. We have gone through the convolutions of supposedly superior scientific method, right up-to-the-minute and beyond, only to end up where intuitive gifts and metaphysical KNOWING took us a long time ago.

BOHM'S BRAVE NEW WORLD

On a final serious note, while writing of the increasingly hazy demarcation between mind perception and so-called objective reality, it is essential to mention David Bohm's holographic universe concept. It is only a metaphor but it is an exciting one and it could well contain the essential truth needed to integrate organic wholeness, what is Divine and the epistemology of perception. The proper union of these three elements of philosophy has eluded scientist and thinkers since the dawn of thinking. How does Bohm's hypothesis help?

Firstly, let me explain an important point about holograms. Everyone knows that you can see them in three dimensions; it is a means of visualizing an object as a volume solid and is used in museums to preserve valuable specimens intact while allowing them to be appreciated by visitors. What is less well known, but is actually a far more important property of holograms, is that each part contains the whole. If you take a pair of scissors and cut a hologram in two, both halves contain the full picture. If you cut it in half again, each new fragment still contains the whole picture. This can go on indefinitely; no matter how small the piece, it still contains the whole image, though obviously is becomes fainter and fainter as the representational elements become smaller and smaller.

Bohm's novel insight was to suppose that physical reality may be constructed in some similar fashion. In other words, the universe itself acts as a hologram. Bohm called the picture we see the explicate order (from explicit); and the hidden total inner picture, the implicate order (from implicit or hidden). What does this actually mean? Well, if Bohm's idea is correct, it means that all parts of existence are contained in each tiny fragment. The desk on which my word-processor stands has all the elements of creation and reality, from the dawn of time to the end of the universe; every atom, every galaxy. If I unscrew one of the drawer handles and inspect it, even THAT could contain the totality of everything! This is an appalling thought but at the same time a thrilling one.

Certain threads from the VIRTUAL MEDICINE paradigm now begin to converge. For example we saw that Sheldrake's morphogenic fields are something super-ordinary; something above the range of energy and matter, that acted as a kind of blueprint. Could these fields be part of the implicate order? If so, does it not mean that DNA, that wonder chemical substance that contains the codes for living organisms, could be the life bridge between the implicate and explicate orders? Remember Roger Coghill's suggestion that the DNA molecule works as a transmitter aerial on page 21. But what does it transmit; radio waves? Or some bolder cosmic message of order and creation.

The mind itself, of course, will form part of that bridge to reality. Information, as I have said before, IMPLIES consciousness and awareness. You can't have one without the other. This is a potential paradox solved by reference to the eastern sages and the British Empiricist philosophers already referred to above: what we are is a product of what we perceive and vice versa. There is no difference between the perceiver and the perceived.

Nobody knows if Bohm's hypothesis is the final answer but in terms of consistency, it is a hard theory to beat, because almost all mysteries of the world we experience become understandable in simple terms of explicit vs. implicit order. Take telepathy or past lives as examples. If all of existence is wrapped up in every little fragment of reality, that would also include the matter inside our brains. Any piece of the brain has the whole of the rest of reality wrapped up in it somewhere (I am purposely side-stepping the fact that mind is unlikely to be exactly congruent with brain). We can potentially know everything, all in an instant. Now that's what ancient sages have been saying, so the idea is not so alien. What is new is a means to understand how this could be true. Bohm's brave new universe is very satisfying in many respects.

The corollary is that, if we know everything, then we have to selectively un-know things, otherwise our consciousness would just go into overdrive and... well, who knows what? We can speculate. Because if knowledge is not merely brain, then perhaps all knowledge is potentially knowable. That sounds as if we would become divine; we could be part of the Source of All Creation.

That, however, must remain the theme for another book.

THE LAST WORD

Let's end on a lighter note by taking *VIRTUAL MEDICINE* to the extreme outer fringe. It has been postulated that man may one day abandon his flesh body and become so integrated with computers that our personality resides entirely within the software of the cyber domain. This would be *VIRTUAL LIVING*, rather than the virtual reality being debated today; consciousness would be in the computer world looking out into what we assume to be reality, instead of the other way round.

Celebrated writer Arthur C. Clarke first put forward this idea in a 1956 book *The City and The Stars*, though how the fictional civilization managed this trick he does not reveal in the story.

But writer Bob Ettinger takes it very seriously and his book *Man Into Superman* is definitely non-fiction. He foresees the day when it will be possible to transfer our human personalities to a software package which thinks, feels and communicates.

We would then dispense with the inconvenient restrictions of the body and its incessant demands for foraging and procreation. Should such a scenario ever come to pass, we would of course be 'immortal', though there would need to be back-up copies for safety. These back-up personalities would have to be updated regularly, otherwise they would become invalid because they were missing too many experiences.

Ed Regis, author of *Great Chicken Mambo and the Transhuman Condition* (which for both our sake's I had better state is subtitled *Science Slightly Over The Edge!*) calls this state post-biological man. You might worry that, even if you felt you were now inside a computer- that you were really there- you would no longer be able to experience anything real. Any input sensations would be mere simulation. Well, according to David Hume, greatest of the British Empiricists referred to above, that's all you ever get in life anyway! All of living is only a mind simulation of whatever is 'out there' (if anything).

It may come as a shock to readers to realize that these ideas are being seriously debated. Do not be tempted to scoff at this possibility of cyber-life. It may be closer than you think. 'What Nature can do,' the late Arthur C. Clarke wrote, 'Man can also do in his own way'.

As Frederik Pohl, also a sci-fi writer, stated in a 1964 Playboy article '*Intimations of Immortality*': 'The essential 'you' isn't your body. It is what we call your personality, your memory, your mind. This essential 'you' could be preserved inside a computer, a collection of magnetic impulses in an IBM machine'.

What then would be the state of *VIRTUAL MEDICINE*?

Presumably physicians like me would have to be computer geeks and know how to handle floppy discs, save, copy, backup, restore and edit files. Illness might then be a question of corrupted memory or glitches and we would have to put this right. A major operation would be to shut down the computer system and re-install you from a backup. By then evolution would be reduced to thinking up newer and better software packages to broadcast ourselves from.

This prospect makes Aldous Huxley's Brave New World seem like a vicarage tea party. But if in the far distant future it came about, and there just happened to be a mouldering centuries-old copy of this book found on a forgotten shelf somewhere, no-one will be able to turn to the end of the last page and read those foolish words:

it could never happen!

(One quick witted reader of the first edition pointed out that the book did in fact end with those very words! Touché!)

Well now it ends with these:

"One would not think that benefactors of humanity would have to run the gauntlet of bigotry, tyranny and oppression - yet except for these few apostles of scientific truth, those great and heroic men who dared to keep their faces toward the light, medicine today would still be in the Dark Ages..."

It's from *Magic, Myth and Medicine* by D. T. Atkinson

"Behind every man now alive stand thirty ghosts, for that is the ratio by which the dead outnumber the living. Since the dawn of time, roughly a hundred billion human beings have walked the planet Earth.

--Now this is an interesting number, for by a curious coincidence there are approximately a hundred billion stars in our local universe, the Milky Way. So for every man [and woman] who has ever lived, in this universe, there shines a star."

(from Arthur C. Clarke's foreword in *2001, A Space Odyssey*, 1968)

Clarke himself, the towering visionary giant of science futures, probably gets a whole galaxy allocated to him!

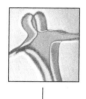

RESOURCES

CHAPTER 1

1 A. Linde, 'The Self-Reproducing Inflationary Universe', *Scientific American* vol 9, no. 1, 1998.

2 M. White, *Isaac Newton, The Last Sorcerer* (Fourth Estate, 1997).

3 R. Sheldrake, *The Rebirth of Nature* (Rider, 1990).

4 J. C. Eccles, *Evolution of the Brain: Creation of the Self* (Routledge, 1989).

5 R. D. Pearson, *Intelligence Behind the Universe* (The Headquarters Publishing Co. Ltd., 1990).

6 R. Gerber, *Vibrational Medicine* (Santa Fe, NM: Bear, 1988).

7 A. Abrams, *New Concepts in Diagnosis and Treatment* (San Francisco: Philopolis Press, 1916).

8 H. Gaier (ed), *Thorsons Encyclopaedic Dictionary of Homeopathy* (Thorsons, 1991).

9 R. O. Becker, *Cross Currents: The Perils of Electropollution, The Promise of Electromedicine* (NY: Tarcher/Putnam, 1990): 239.

10 J. R. Thomas, J. Schrot and A. Liboff, 'Production of passive behaviour in mice by means of lithium cyclotron resonance', *Biomagnetics* 7 (1986): 349.

CHAPTER 2

1 H. Schiegl, *Healing Magnetism* (Century, 1987): 13.

2 H. S. Burr, *Blueprint for Immortality* (Saffron Walden: C W Daniel and Co, 1972).

3 Ibid.

4 G. Lakhovsky, *The Secret of Life* (True Health Publishing Co, 1951 [English translation copyright 1970 by Mark Clement]): 3.

5 Ibid.

6 K. Mumby, *The Complete Guide to Allergy and Environmental Illness* (Thorsons, 1993).

7 A. Nodon, 'Les nouvelles radiations ultra-pénétrantes et à cellule vivante', *Revue Scientifique* 22nd October 1927: 609.

8   Lakhovsky, op cit. 111.

9   R. O. Becker, *The Body Electric* (Morrow, New York 1985).

10 J. L. Oschman, 'What Is Healing Energy? Part 2: Measuring the Fields of Life', *Journal of Bodywork and Movement Therapies* January 1997: 117–22.

11 R. Sheldrake, *New Science of Life* (Rider, 1990).

12. Watson L, Lifetide, Corotnet edition, 1990, London, pp. 173-75

13. B Josephson, November 1981 issue of BRAIN MIND BULLETIN: (regarding an editorial from NATURE.

CHAPTER 3

1   Chang Tsai, quoted in Fung Yu-lan, *A Short History of Chinese Philosophy* (NY: Macmillan, 1958): 279.

2   Sir T. Lewis, 'The Nocifensor System of Nerves and its Reactions', *British Medical Journal* 27th February 1937: 431.

3   P. de Vernejoul *et al.*, 'Etude Des Méridiens D'Acupuncture par les Traceurs Radioactifs', *Bull. Acad. Natle. Med.* vol. 169 (22nd October, 1985): 1071—5.

4   R. O. Becker, *Cross Currents: The Perils of Electropollution, The Promise of Electromedicine* (NY: Tarcher/Putnam, 1990): 90.

5   H. Motoyama, *Theories of the Chakras* (IL: Theosophical Publishing House, 1981).

6   Hunt Dr. V, Massey W, Weinberg R, Bruyere R, and Hahn P., *'Project Report, A Study of Structural Integration from Neuromuscular, Energy Field and Emotional Approches.'* U.C.L.A., 1977.

7   D. J. Matzke, 'Prediction: Future Electronics Will Be Disrupted due to Consciousness', paper at *Towards a Science of Consciousness* conference, Tucson II, University of Arizona, 1996.

8   J. R. Wosley, *Everyone's Guide to Acupuncture* (Cassell, 1973): 43.

9   Ibid: 44.

10 M. Wexu, *The Ear, Gateway to Balancing the Body: A Modern Guide to Acupuncture* (NY: ASI Publishers, 1975).

11 A.G. Gurwitsch: "Über Ursachen der Zellteilung". Arch. Entw. Mech. Org. 51 (1922), 383-415

12 F. A. Popp, 'New Avenues in Medicine' (two-part radio broadcast in the series *Neues Aus Kultur und Wissenschaft*; Deutschlandfunk Radio, Aug–Sept 1979. Published in H Brügemann (ed), *Bioresonance and Multiresoance Therapy* (vol 1; Haug: Brussels, 1990

13 F. A. Popp et al., Experientia 44, 543 (1988).

14 F. A. Popp et al., Recent Advances in Biophoton Research and its Applications, eds. F. A. Popp et al., World Scientific, Singapore, 1992.

15 Fröhlich H, 1988. *Theoretical Physics and Biology*. In: Fröhlich H (Ed.) *Biological Coherence and Response to External Stimuli*. Berlin: Springer-Verlag, 1- 24.

16 Smith C W, Is a living system a macroscopic quantum system? Frontier Perspectives, 7(1), 9- 15 (1988)

CHAPTER 4

1 Stortebecker P. *Dental Caries as a Cause of Nervous Disorders*, Bio-Probe Inc, Orlando, USA, 1986. P. 39.

2 R. Voll, 'The Phenomenon of Medicine Testing in Electroacupuncture According to Voll', *Am Acupunct* 8, 1980: 97–104.

3 K.-G. Chen, 'Applying Quantum Interference to EDST Medicine Testing', *IEEE Engineering in Medicine and Biology* (four-part series) May/June 1996: 64–6.

4 J Benveniste, 'The Memory of Molecules', *The Independent* Friday Review, 19th March 1999.

5 J. J. Tsuei, C. W. Lehman, F. Lam Jr, D. Zhu, 'A Food Allergy Study Utilizing the EAV Acupuncture Technique', *Am J Acupunct* 12, 1984: 105–16.

6 P. Chou, J. J. Tsuei, C. H. Chen, 'Clinical Application of Bioenergy in the Cardiovascular System', report to the ROC National Research Institute of Chinese Medicine, 1985: NRICM-84–103.

7 Dr Julian Kenyon, personal communication June 1998, in the form of a draft chapter of a forthcoming book.

CHAPTER 5

1 Noma News, Newsletter 7, Southampton, July 1999, pp. 11- 32

2. Clark H R, *The Cure for All Cancers*,

3. J. Kenyon, *21st Century Medicine* (Thorsons, 1986).

4. R. Van Wijk and F. A. C. Wilegart, 'Homeopathic Remedies and Pressure-induced Changes in Galvanic Resistance of the Skin', Dept of Molecular Biology, State University of Utrecht, Research Unit for Complementary Medicine, Padualaan 8, 3584 CH Utrecht, 1989.

5 R. Van Wijk, 'Homeopathic Medicines in Closed Phials Tested by Changes in the Conductivity of the Skin: A Critical Evaluation. Blind Testing and Partial Elucidation of the Mechanisms', Dept of Molecular Biology, State University of Utrecht, Research Unit for Complementary Medicine, Padualaan 8, 3584 CH Utrecht, 1992.

6 D. J. Matzke, 'Prediction: Future Electronics Will Be Disrupted due to Consciousness', paper at *Towards a Science of Consciousness* conference, Tucson II, University of Arizona, 1996.

7   Lawden DF, Separability of Psycho-physical Systems, Psycho-Energet-
ics. The Journal of Psycho-physical Systems, vol 4, no 1, 1-10 (1981).

CHAPTER 6
1   E. Rasche, *Elektronische Homeopathie* (Friesenheim: Medtronik
Trading GmbH, 1998).
2   H. Gaier (ed), *Thorsons Encyclopaedic Dictionary of Homeopathy*
(Thorsons, 1991): 57
3   Quoted in H. Brügemann (ed), *Bioresonance and Multiresonance
Therapy* (vol 1; Haug: Brussels, 1990 [English edn, 1993]).
4   Rasche, op cit
5   Brügemann, op cit

CHAPTER 7
1   E. Hamlyn, *The Healing Art of Homeopathy* (The Organon of Samuel
Hahnemann, Beaconsfield Publishers, 1979).
2   L. Watson, *Supernature* (Hodder and Stoughton, 1973).
3   Davenas E, Benveniste J et al. 'Human basophil degranulation triggered
by very dilute antiserum against IgE, *Nature 333* (1988):816; 1988..
4   H.-H. Reckeweg, *Homotoxicology – illness and healing through anti-
homotoxic therapy* (Albuquerque, NM: Menaco Publishing Co, 1980).
5   A. Pischinger, *Matrix and Matrix Regulation, Basis for a Holistic
Theory in Medicine* (Brussels: Haug International, 1986).
6   H. Gaier (ed), *Thorsons Encyclopaedic Dictionary of Homeopathy*
(Thorsons, 1991): 66.
7   S. Bawin and W. R. Adey, 'First report of ELF fields producing calcium
efflux from nerve cells', *Proceedings of the National Academy of Sciences* 73 (1976): 1999.
8   Personal communication from George Burns, Manchester homeopath.
9   Gaier, op cit: 345.
10 K Mumby, *The Allergy Handbook* (Thorsons, 1989).
11 E Bach and F J Wheeler, *The Bach Flower Remedies* (New Canaan,
CT: Keats, 1977).
12 E. Rasche, *Elektronische Homeopathie* (Friesenheim: Medtronik
Trading GmbH, 1998).
13 M. Bastide, M. Doucet Jaboeuf, V. Daurat. Activity and chrono-
pharmacology of very low doses of physiological immune inducers,
Immunology Today (6:234-235) 1985.
14 B.J. Youbicier-Simo, F. Boudard, M. Mekaouche, M. Bastide, J.D.
Baylé. Effects of embryonic bursectomy and in ovo administration of

highly diluted bursin on a adrenocorticotropic and immune response to chickens. *International Journal of Immunotherapy* (IX:169-180) 1993.

15 P.C. Endler, W. Pongratz, G. Kastberger, F.A.C. Wiegant, J. Schulte The effect of highly diluted agitated thyroxine of the climbing activity of frogs. *Veterinary and Human Toxicology* (36:56-59) 1994.

16 P.C. Endler, W. Pongratz, R. van Wijk, K. Waltl, H. Hilgers, R. Brandmaier, Transmission of hormone information by non-molecular means. *FASEB Journal* (8:A400(abs)) 1995 .

17 F. Senekowitsch, P.C.Endler, W. Pongratz, C.W. Smith, Hormone effects by CD record/replay. *FASEB Journal* (9: A392(abs)) 1995.

18 E. del Giudice, G. Preparata, G. Vitiello, Water as a free electric dipole laser. *Physical Reviews Letter* (61:1085-1088) 1988, .

19 J Benveniste, 'The Memory of Molecules', *The Independent* Friday Review, 19th March 1999.

CHAPTER 8

1 K. Mumby, *The Allergy Handbook* (Thorsons, 1989).

2. Ostrander S and Schroeder L, Super-Learning 2000, Souvenir Press, London, 1995, pp. 210- 211.

3. Stortebecker P. Dental Caries as a Cause of Nervous Disorders, Bio-Probe Inc, Orlando, USA, 1986. p73.

4 J. Diamond and L. W. Cowden, *The Alternative Medicine Definitive Guide to Cancer* (Tiburon, CA: Future Medicine Publishing Inc., 1997): 1027.

CHAPTER 9

1 Szent-Gyorgi, Introduction to a Sub-Moledular Biology, *Academic Press*, New York, 1960.

2 Berezin Martinez, Artificial Light-Sensitive Enzyme Systems as Chemical AMplifiers of Weak Light Signals, *Photochemistry Photobiology .29*, March 1979, pp637-650.

3 J Liberman Light: Medicine of the Future, Bear and Co, Santa Fe, 1991, p51.

4 Beral V, et al.,'Malignant melanoma and exposure to fluorescent light' Lancet 2 (1982) pp 290-292.

5 B. Bhattacharya, *Gem Therapy* (Calcutta: Firma KLM Private Ltd, 1993).

6 T. Engineer, P. Richards, 'VRIC Imaging the Photon', paper presented at the International Forum of New Science, Denver, Colorado, 1997.

7 T. Engineer, 'Biolumanetics – The Science of Life-Light', *Positive Health* March 1998: 23–7.

8. http://square.umin.ac.jp/mtnet/E/meridiantest.html, as downloaded 25th August 2004, 15.00 Pacific Time.

CHAPTER 10

1　Lovelock JE, *Gaia A new look at life on Earth*, Oxford University Press, 1979

2. R. O. Becker, *Cross Currents: The Perils of Electropollution, The Promise of Electromedicine* (NY: Tarcher/Putnam, 1990): 182.

3　K. Mumby, *The Complete Guide to Food Allergy and Environmental Illness* (Thorsons, 1993): 193.

4　Ibid: 69.

5　R. Coghill, *Something in the Air* (Coghill Research Laboratories, Lower Race, Gwent NP4 5UH, Wales, 1997).

6　Dr B. Kohler, 'The Basic Principles of Multiresonance Therapy with Biologically Effective Environmental Signals', in H Brügemann (ed), *Bioresonance and Multiresoance Therapy* (vol 1; Haug: Brussels, 1990 [English edn 1993]).

7　K. Mumby, *The Allergy Handbook* (Thorsons, 1989).

8　Becker, op cit: 302.

9　J. Pawlik, P. Chase, *Newcastle Guide to Healing with Crystals* (North Hollywood, CA: Newcastle Publishing Co, 1988).

10 Mumby, op cit.

CHAPTER 11

1. You may find useful clues in this very disjointed story from the ISTA website: http://www.scenartech.com

2. 1: Usp Fiziol Nauk. 2001 Jul-Sep;32(3):79-86 (article in Russian)

3. Travell J G and Simons D, Myofascial Pain and Dysfunction: The Trigger Point Manual, vols 1 and 2. see also Wikipedia:
http://en.wikipedia.org/wiki/Trigger_point

4. Personal communication, Oct 2007

CHAPTER 12

1　J. D. Beck, S. Offenbacher, R. Williams, P. Gibbs and R. Garcia, 'Peri-odontitis: A Risk Factor for Coronary Heart Disease?', *Annals of Peri-odontology* vol. 3, no. 1, July 1998: 127–41.

2　Stortebecker P. Dental Caries as a Cause of Nervous Disorders, Bio-Probe Inc, Orlando, USA, 1986. P74.

3　Stortebecker P. Dental Caries as a Cause of Nervous Disorders, Bio-Probe Inc, Orlando, USA, 1986. P34.

4　Ibid: p.116.

5 R. Turk, 'Iatrogenic Damage Due to High-speed Drilling', paper presented at the Scientific Session at the dedication of the Princeton Bio Center, New Jersey, 13th June, 1981.

6 H. Raue, 'Resistance to Therapy; Think of Tooth Fillings', *Medical Practice* vol 32, no 72, 6th September 1980: 2303—9.

7 J. E. Bouquot, *In Review of Nico, G V Black's Forgotten Disease*, The Maxillofacial Centre, 583 Tibbs Rd, Morgantown, West Virginia, Third Edition, 1995.

8 G. Meinig, *Root Canal Cover-up* (Ojai, CA: Bion Publishing, 1995).

9 Radio interview of the *Laura Lee Show*, transcript published in the *Townsend Letter for Doctor and Patient* August/September 1996.

CHAPTER 13

1. Proton magnetic resonance at very low levels in the ambient field caused sub-capsular cataracts in bovine eye lenses.

2. Lysozyme effects on Micrococcus lysodeikticus was shown to be nutrition-sensitive in the conditions for magnetic resonance and solutions had "memory".

(Fröhlich H, 1988 Theoretical Physics and Biology. In: Fröhlich, H (Ed.) Biological Coherence and Response to External Stimuli. Berlin: Springer-Verlag, 1- 24

3. http://www.i-sis.org.uk/ No 15 Summer 2002

4. L. Rey, Thermoluminescence of ultra-high dilutions of lithium chloride and sodium chloride, Physica A 323 (2003), pp. 67–74.

5. Issue 2399 of New Scientist magazine, 14 June 2003, page 22

6. 1996 Modulation of human neutrophil activation by "electronic" phorbol myristate acetate (PMA) Federation of American Societies for Experimental Biology Journal (10:A1479(abs)) Y Thomas, H Litime, J Benveniste

7. 1997 Transatlantic transfer of digitized antigen signal by telephone link. Journal of Allergy and Clinical Immunology (99:S175 (abs.) J. Benveniste, P. Jurgens, W. Hsueh, J. Aïssa.

8. FASEB Journal, 1999, vol. 13, p. A852

CHAPTER 14

1. Meek G W, "After We Die, What Then?" Ariel Press, 1987, Columbus, Ohio, pp. 153- 165

2. http://www.worlditc.org/ (accessed 04/12/08 at 19.15 PDT)

3- 5 *Ibid.*

6. Raudive K, *"Breakthrough"*, Taplinger, New York, 1971, p. 15

7. Meek G W, *Ibid.*

8. Spiricom booklet, study it on-line here:
    http://www.worldic.org/h_07_meek_spiri_000_007.htm

9. Rogo, D S, *"Phone Calls From The Dead"*, Prentice-Hall, Englewood Cliffs, NJ, 1979

10. Watson L, *"The Secret Life of Inanimate Objects"*, Destiny Books, Rochster VT, 1992, pp. 206-7

11. Peasboro J, *"The Devil in the Machine: Is your computer possessed by a demon?"* unable to find the real publisher, though there is reference to it all over the Web.

CHAPTER 15

1. Dr Julian Kenyon, personal communication in the form of a draft chapter for a book on, bio-energtic medicine, October 1998.

2. Quoted in G. Zukav, *The Dancing Wu-Li Masters*

3. Maby, Proceedings of the Scientific and Technical Congress of radionics and Radiesthesia 1950. Prof. Chauvin, Znanie-Sila magazine No. 9, 1967

4. Tiller, WA 'A gas discharge device for investigating Focussed Human Intention' Journal of Scientific Exploration Vol.4 No.2 (The American group is headed by M. Sue Benford RN MA President of PreComp Inc. and Public Health Information Services Inc., Ohio.)

5. D. J. Matzke, 'Prediction: Future Electronics Will Be Disrupted due to Consciousness', paper at *Towards a Science of Consciousness*, Tucson II, University of Arizona, 1996.

6. M. Talbot, *The Holographic Universe* (HarperCollins, 1996).

7. R. C. W. Ettinger, *Man Into Superman* (NY: St Martin's Press, 1972).

8. E. Regis, *Great Mambo Chicken and the Transhuman Condition* (Penguin Science, 1992).

7   Quoted in Regis, op cit.

INDEX

Abrams, Albert 6–9, 11–12, 64, 94, 130, 166, 171
accident 127–8
accompanying remedies 141
acidosis 192–4, 200
Acupro 127, 139, 141, 150
acupuncture 27
meridians see meridians
see also electro-acupuncture
acupuncture points 25–6
in Kirlian photography 49
and skin resistance 54, 69
and Vega testing 75
Voll system 54–9, 55, 87, 95–6, 133–4
addictions 99–100
Adey, W. Ross 120
Adey Window 120
alcohol, quality improvement 97–8
Allen, Henry C. 124
allergies:
and aura 88
causal chains 145–6
as information field effects 66, 97
instant reactions 131
and MORA machine 97
phenolic compounds 83–6
vaccination cause 121–2, 146
allergy testing:
using ACR 51
using EAV 66–7
AMI scanner 40–2, 71–2
amplifiers 75, 79
anaesthesia 39

animal experiments 94–5
animal magnetism 18–19
antibiotics 203
antioxidants 199–200
Arndt-Schulz's Law 25, 119–20, 121, 219
arthritis 209, 213
Attila von Szalay 239
aura glasses 44
auras 1, 44–5
and Rolfing 44–5
auriculo-acupuncture 49–51
auriculo-cardiac reflex (ACR) 51
Avatar 139, 141, 144
Avogradro number 218
Ayurvedic gem elixir therapy 157–8, 164–5
Ayurvedic tradition 39–43

Bacci, Marcello 239
Bach, Dr Edward 118, 125–6
Bach Flower Remedies 118, 125–8, 140
Bachler, Kathe 182
bacillus "X" (BX) 231
bacillus "Y" (BY) 231
band pass devices 101–4
Bangor University 229
Barr, Sir James 9
Basic Therapy, in BRT 95
Baule, Gerhard 29
Becker, Prof Robert O. 12, 25–8, 38–9, 176–8, 184
Benveniste, Prof Jacques 67, 104, 112, 130–1, 144, 222, 230

benzene poisoning 148–9
Ber, Dr Abram 85
Bergson, Henri 3
Berkeley, George 89
BHI 168
BICOM 93, 101–4, 235
Billings, Dr 213
bio-battery 145
bio-plasmic body 44, 48–9
biological age 79–80,
biological energy 1
biological radiation 21–3
biological receptors 131
biological resonance 11–15
Biolumanetics 166–9
biomagnetic fields 29
biomagnetics 27
Biomed 139
biophotons 51
bioresonance therapy (BRT) 91–106
Black, G.V. 211
blockages 36, 100
body consciousness 38–9
body cycles 60
light energy radiation treatment 156–65
semi-conductor role 25
Bohm, David 268–70
bound water 39
Boyd, Dr William 10–11, 64, 94
Brahman (ultimate reality) 39
brain:
in Bohm's hypothesis 270
magnetic field, exterior

extension 26, 29
brain magneto-gram 29
brainwave patterns 161–2
BRT see bioresonance
    therapy
Bregemann, Hans 101,
    104, 105
Bruyere, Rosalyn 45
Burr, Prof Harold Saxton
    19–20, 38, 48

Caduceus II 156–65
calibration 74
California Essences 128
cancer:
    EDS preventive treat-
        ment 149–51
    and infective foci 147
    MORA treatment 100–1
    Multiple Wave Oscilla-
        tor treatment 23
    oscillatory disequilib-
        rium factor 22–3
    and soil types 20–1
Candida 124
capacitance 69
Capra, Fritjof vii, 262
causal chains 145–7
Cayce, Edgar 145
cells:
    and biological radiation
        21–3, 96, 116
    death flash 155
    semi-conductor role 25
Central Measurement
    Points (CMPs) 59, 61,
    95–6
and electro-dermal com-
    puter screening 133–4,
    133
chakras 39–43, 41
    light treatment 163–4
Chaplin, Martin 220
Chen, Dr Kuo-Gen 65
Ch'i 34–5, 39, 46–7
Ch'i detectors 46–7
Ch'i generators 46–7
Chigung 46

children 99
chronic disease, layers
    221
Clark, James Hoyte 138
Clarke, Arthur C. 263
Clinic-in-a-Case 139
clockwork universe
    concept 3
CMPs see Central Meas-
    urement Points
Cobain, Kurt (computer
    ghost) 247
Coghill, Roger 21, 131,
    178–80, 269
Cohen, David 28, 29
coherent light 154, 166
collagen fibres, as merid-
    ian channels 38
colour, biological effects
    153–4
complex homeopathy
    (German system)
    113–15, 143–4,
computers 179
conductance 69
connective tissue matrix
    25, 116–17
consciousness 5
    definition 6
    and evolution 31
    and observer effect 88,
        241
Cook, Vauhgn 144
cooked teeth 204–5
cranium, infection in
    brain 202–3
Crile, Dr George 24–5
crowns, dental 202
crystals 158, 185–6
Curry Grid 181
cyclotron resonance
    12–14, 225

database, in electro-der-
    mal computer screen-
    ing 135–8
DC body field 25, 38
de-differentiation 25

degenerative diseases 214
dentistry 201–16
    x-rays 179
    see also mercury dental
        fillings
Dermatron 53, 66, 85
detox programmes 82
diagnosis:
    through aura 44–5
    before symptoms see
        prognosis
    in electro-dermal com-
        puter screening 135–8
    with the Emanometer
        10
    information fields in
        148
    through Kirlian photo-
        graphy 49
    percussion method 7, 10
    using ACR 51
    using the Reflexophone
        7–8
diatherapuncteur 53
Digibio(.com) 227
digital biology 222
digital pocket recorder
    (ghost hunting) 255
dilution see potentization
direct light enhancement
    94
disease:
    definition 5
    electromagnetic signals
        of 91–4
    energetic view 21–2
    humoral nature 115
disintegrative psychosis
    165
disorder control 74, 75,
    79, 86
DNA 21, 131, 238–9
Dong Chen 47
drainage remedies 117,
    119, 199
Drown, Ruth 11
dynamic energies 92

ear acupuncture 49–51, 223

Earth energies see Gaia

EAV method 58–9, 87, 94

Einthoven, Willem 29

electrical equipment 178–80

electrical fields, in teeth 207–8

electricity, in the home/ office 177–80

electro-acupuncture 38, 53–71

Voll method see EAV

electro-cardiography 29

electro-dermal computer screening 133–51

electro-dermal screening 65, 138–43

electro-homeopathy 129

electronic voice phenomena (EVP) 238–256

electro-pollution 176

electromagnetic fields: in allergy sufferers 88

Earth's 171–6

electromagnetic radiation: environmental 23–4

and imprinting 129–30

electromagnetic resonance 12

electromagnetic signals (EMS), of disease 91–4

of substances 221

electronic gem therapy 160–4

electrotherapy 27

ELF radiation 14, 174, 177, 181

Emanometer 10–11, 65, 94

emotions, measurement 19

EMP from nuclear weapons 184–5

endocrine glands, potentized support signals 144

energy being, life as 15–16

energy healing 12

energy medicine 5–6

three categories 26–7

energy readings: at acupuncture points 56–7

negative factors 60

energy transference 17

Energy-reinforcement Techniques 27

Engineer, Thrity 168–9

ENT problems 125

environmental pollution 196

enzymes, potentized support signals 143

EPFX 256

Ernst, Edzard, Prof 221

essential fatty acids, potentized support signals 143

Ettinger, Bob 271

explicate order 269

extra-cellular fluid (ECF) 190–1

extrasensory perception 12

extremely-low-frequency (ELF) fields 14, 174, 177, 181

eyes, light transmission role 156–7

faith healing 15

field effects 20

filters: in electro–dermal screening 140–1

in Vega testing 77–8, 80, 104

Fishbein, Morris 233

Flower Essence Society 128

flu, as stroke cause 129, 142–3, 146

foci 62–3, 147, 205

teeth 208–15

food: phenolic compounds in 83–6

vital energy in 49

FT-ICE mass spectrometer 218

Gaia 171–86

Gaikin, Dr M.K. 48 221

gall stones (fake) 82

Gardiner, Dr Robert 83

"gating" (Rife method) 235

GB-4000 (device) 235

gem elixir therapy 157–8, 164–5

gem therapy 156–65

gems, effects 159, 160–1, 185–6

genetic toxins 123–5

geomagnetic field see magnetosphere

geopathic stress 172, 220

filters 77–8

Gerber, Dr Richard 6

Ghosts, see video ghosts

grids 181–2

gum disease 201, 216

Gurwitsch, Alexander 154

Hahn, Dr 206

Hahnemann, Samuel 108–9, 113, 123–4

Hartman Net 181

healers, magnetic field generation 15, 48

healing 4–5, 251–3

and electromagnetic resonance 12

hands-on 17

in Kirlian photography 48

heart, magnetic field 29

heavy metal poisoning 206–7

HEEL 168

heredity 123–5

Hering, Constantine 117

Hering's Law 117–8
heterodyning 229
High-energy Transfer
    Techniques 27
history 17–31
Hoffman, Samuel O. 8
holographic universe
    concept 257–9
homeopathy 27, 107–23
    Arndt-Schulz low-dose
    law 25, 119–20, 121,
    219
    complex 113–15, 143–4,
    201
    electronic 91
    remedies:
    in complex homeopathy
    113–15, 143–4
    testing 10
    homeostasis 121
    foci disturbance 62
    and Vega testing 75–6
Homotoxicology 115,
    117
homotoxicosis 116
Horder, Sir Thomas 10
hormones, potentized
    support signals 144
Hoyland, Philip 233
human energy field 88
Hume, David 271
Hunt, Dr Valerie 45
Hunter, Dr William 202
Huxley, Aldous 272
hypertension study 68–9
hypnosis 26
hypothalamic disorder
    61–2

immune system 188
    dentistry effects 204
    radiation effects 176–8
implicate order 269
imponderables 144
imprinting 128–30, 140
Indicator Drops 57, 61,
    66–7, 73, 86, 96, 134
infertility 99

information fields 4–5,
    30, 48
    in allergy testing 52
    in diagnosis 148
    effects: allergy 66, 97
Internet, healing over,
    explanation 130–1
interstitial fluid 115–16
ionizing radiation 182–4
isopathy 113–15

Josephson, Brian 28–9
Juergenson, Friedrich 241,
    256
jungle diseases 149

Kanzius 236
Katz, Richard 128
Kay, Prof Barry 9
Kemeny, Prof Janos 189
Kenyon, Dr Julian 51,
    71–2, 87, 145, 259
Khronos, Dr Yuri 47
Kilner, Dr Walter 44
Kilner screen 44
kinesiology 87
Kirlian photography 22,
    47–9, 72
Kirlian, Semyon D. 47
Klass, Dr Jeffrey 197–9
Koenig, Hans Otto 248
Kronner, Fritz 204
kundalini, electronic
    257-72

L-Field (Field of Life) 20,
    44, 48, 66
Lachesis (remedy) 219
Lakhovsky, Georges 20–4,
    91, 96, 116, 223
Lasers 168
Lawden, Prof D.F. 88–9
Lewis, Sir Thomas 37, 51
Liberman, Jacob 158
Lieber, Douglas 150
light therapy 153–69

Limbic Ark 228- 30
Linde, Prof Andrei 2
LISTEN system 138, 139,
    148–9
lithium experiment 14,
    114
liver cleanse 81–2
living universe theories 5
Lovelock, Richard 171
low light frequencies 94
Lumanetics 167
Luminator 166–9
Lux Caduceus II 156–65
lymphocytes, energy field
    effects 217–8

McFee, Richard 29
Macy, Mark (INIT) 251
Maddox, Sir John 112
magnetic reversals 175–6
magnetic-resonance imag-
    ing (MRI) 12–13, 27
magneto-encephalogram
    (MEG) 29
magnetosphere 172, 173,
    175
mal-illumination 155–6
masking, energetic 75–6
Maslow, Abram 5
matrix 115–17, 199
    and cell vibrations 21–3,
    96, 116
matter 4–5, 22, 35
Mayo Clinic 218
Meek, George W. 242
Meinig, George 216
MeniSre's disease 208
mercury dental fillings
    98, 104, 207–9, 208
meridians 37–8
    in acupuncture 25–6
    and Ch'i 34–6
    CMPs 59
    correlations 57–9
    energy readings 56–7
    Indicator Drop 57
    and teeth 210–12
Mersmann, Ludger 92

mesenchyme therapy 79, 115–18, 193, 199
Mesmer, Anton 18–19
miasm 123–5
milieu int,rieur 188–9, 192
Miller method 67, 141
mind-brain link 88
mineralization 196–7, 200
minerals, potentized support signals 143
Minimal Energy Techniques 26
minimum dose 119–21
mobile phones 179, 218
monkeys, 100 effect 31
MORA firm 139
MORA machine 92–8, 100–2, 128
Morell, Dr Franz 91–2, 128, 227
morphogenic fields 30–1, 48, 258
mortal oscillatory rate (MOR) 232
Motoyama, Hiroshi 40–2, 71
Mueller, George J. (ghost) 237
multiple sclerosis 203
Multiple Wave Oscillator 23
muscle injury 164–5

nadis 40
Neafsey, Patricia 121
Nebel, Antoine 124
Neo Bio–Electronic Test 79
Nelson, Bill 229
nerve channels 62–3, 147
neuralgia 211–12
neuro-transmitters, potentized support signals 144
neutralisation 67, 86, 141
Newton, Isaac 3
NICO (neuralgia-inducing cavitational osteonecrosis) 211–3
nocifensor system 37, 51
Nodon, Albert 21–2, 96
Nogier, Dr Paul 49–51
nosodes 117, 118–23
nuclear magnetic-resonance 218
see also magnetic-resonance imaging

observer effect 88, 137
Oersted, Hans Christian 29
operator intrusion 12, 86–7
organ clock concept 36
organ therapies 80–1
organs, stressed:
finding 73, 76–7
most stressed organ concept 57, 76, 77, 80–1
orientation, and electromagnetic resonance 7, 14, 171–2
ortho-immune programme 151
Oscilloclast 8, 10, 65, 94
Ott, John Nash 155, 158
overdosing 119–20
Oxenbaum, Harold 121

Pacific Flower Remedies 128
pain 100–1
Paracelsus 17–18
parasympathetic dominant state 60
past lives 43, 253, 259
peanuts, Aflatoxin on 89–90
Pearson, David 5
Peasboro, Rev. Jim 246
phenolic testing 83–6
pineal gland 156
Pischinger, Prof Alfred 115, 116
plants:
cancer experiment 23, 23
light experiments 154–5
relationships with humans 169
plasma waves 181
PM 2000 76
Pohl, Frederik 271
polarity 219–20
Pope Pius XII 239
Popp, Fritz 51
potentization 109–13
practitioner, health of 74–5
prana 39
Price, Weston 201, 213, 214–15
probe, use 86, 87, 141
prognosis 19, 24, 35, 69–70
progressive vicariation 117
psychokinetic effect 86–7

QSAR (quantitive structure activity relationship 224
quandrant measurement 60–1
quantum science 35, 88–9, 254
Qigung (see Chigung)

rabies 70–71
Rackham, Karen 66
radiation:
artificial 176–80
biological 21–3
Earth-generated 180–3
ionizing 182–4
radiesthesia 11
radioactivity 182–4
radionics 11, 103
Rasche, Erich 92, 94
Raudive, Konstantin 241
Raue, Dr Helmut 208
Ravitz, Dr Leonard 19
reactive oxygen species (ROM) 222
receptors, biological 131

Reckeweg, Dr Hans-Heinrich 115, 116–18
recovery, stages 117–18
Reflexophone 7–9
Regis, Ed 261
regressive vicariation 117, 118
Reichmanis, Maria 25
relationships, interpersonal 167–9
remedies:
  homeopathic see homeopathy, remedies
  imprinting in 128–9, 140
  of non-disease modality 143–4
  and VRIC 166–7
remedy evaluation 63–6, 92
  with Reflexophone 8
remedy filters 80
Rescue Remedy 126
resonance 4, 11–12, 144
  and healing 15
  and water 112
retinograms 29
Rey, Louis (chemist) 220
Richards, Patrick 166, 167
Richardson, Stan 70, 96
"Rife machines" 232
Rife Ray Machine 235
Rife, Royal Raymond 228
Rife "Universal Microscope" 236
right-and-left-brain-coherence 168
Roberts, John 201
Rogo, D. Scott 244
Rolf, Dr Ida P. 45
Rolfing 44–5
root canal fillings 212–14
Rubbia, Carlo 4

SAD (Seasonal Affective Disorder) 154
Sanskrit, 262
samadhi 160, 163
SCENAR (self–controlled

energo-neuro-adaptive regulation) devices 187-200
Schimmel, Helmut 73–4, 77, 78, 79, 86
Schramm, Dr Erwin 79
Schumann waves 180–1
science, naivety in 1–6
scorched hand prints 96
Scott-Morley, Anthony 90, 150
segmental electrogram (SEG) 72
semi–conductors, in body 25
Seven Bach Nosodes 118
shamans 1, 17, 251
Sheldrake, Rupert 3, 30–31, 48, 269
shunomatism 17, 45
sick building syndrome 181
similars, law of 108–9
similimum 114–15
Sinclair, Upton 9
Smith, Cyril 102
Smithells, Ann 148–9
soil types, and cancer 20–1
solar wind 172, 173
son, loss of 169
Soundblaster (card) 221
sound vibrations 177–8
specificity 121–3
spin 12, 42–3
Spiricom (device) 242
spontaneous radiographs 22, 96
SQUID magnetometer 15, 28–30
Stellar Delux (device) 155
Stortebecker, Patrick 62, 147, 202–4
stress:
  de-differentiation effects 25
  lifespan effects 121
  and spin-reversal 42
  in unmasking 75–6
stroke 129, 142–3
substances, non-material

nature of 217-222
sun, radiation from 173–4
sunlight 155–6
sunspots 20, 48, 174–5
symptoms, treating 146–7
Szent-Gyorgi, Albert 153

Tai Ch'i 46
Tai-Ch'i T'u (Supreme Ultimate) 34, 34
tanks, holding 139–40
Tantrism 17
Tao vii, 33
teeth 203–18
telepathy 12, 43
telephone:
  diagnosis over 9
  "ghost" voices over 244
  healing over, explanation 130–1
therapies, categorization 107
thought machines 264–5
thought potentials 88
Tiller, Prof William A. 68–9, 256
Ting points 59, 72
tissues see body tissues
torsion fields 43
Traditional Chinese Medicine (TCM) 33–4
trans–cutaneous nerve stimulation (TENS) 27
trees 19
trigeminal nerve 62–3
Tsuei, Julia J. 67–8
tunnelling 29
Tunnels of Time project 43, 264
Turing, Alan 255
Turk, Ralph 204

vaccinations 121–2, 146
Van Allen belts 172, 173, 175
Van Wijk, R. 87
Vannier, Leon 124

Vega probe 86, 87
vegatest 73–90, 145
Vega Select 168
Vernejoul, Pierre de 37
veterinary bioresonance 95
vibrational medicine see Energy Medicine
video "ghosts" 248
Vimy, Dr 206
virtual living 268-70
Visocekas, Raphael 220
visualization, creative 26
Vitalism viii, 2–3, 175
vitamins, potentized support signals 143
Vo-Cal 360, 255
Voll, Dr Reinhold 53–9,

63–4, 73, 166, 213
Voll meridians see acupuncture points, Voll system
voltage potential 20
VRIC (visual reference of image coherence) 166–9

war of energies 21, 91
Warr, George de la 11
water:
  bound 38
  information properties 110–13, 129, 219
  potentized 164–5
Webster, Ken (poltergeist

affair) 245
West, Ken 168
Whale, Jon 156–9, 163, 164
Williams, Sam, Jr 61
withdrawal symptoms 99
women, angry pelvis in 62, 204
Wright, Payling 63

x-rays 179, 183

Zimmerman, John 28
zonal contact massage 224
Zukav, Gary 262

We hope you enjoyed reading Dr. Keith's amazing writings. There's lots more to discover from him!

You should consider signing up for his monthly subscription newsletter. It's just $59.95 a year and is the best there is. No padding; just plain hard health facts, presented in his inimitable, comprehensive style.

YOU CAN ENROLL HERE:

www.wholesomelivingletter.com

Don't forget to visit his other sites:

www.alternative-doctor.com (main information resource)

www.askdoctorkeith.com (amazing free teleseminars on topics from Virtual Medicine and many other places but you need to enroll - just give your first name and e-mail, that's all)

www.alternative-doctor-radio.com (lots of podcast recordings from radio shows etc)

www.dietwisebook.com
"Diet Wise" Surprising ways that foods can really hurt you! (the best book there is on dieting; it's the book missing from the market that tells you why all set diet plans fail on most people and how to work out what you should be eating.

www.healing-devices.com
A blog based around healing machines like the kind you have been reading about in this book.